PSYCHOSIS AND
THE TRAUMATISED SELF

Psychosis and the Traumatised Self explores what it is like to experience psychosis for individuals with histories of childhood physical and sexual abuse.

The book additionally explores how meaning expressed in psychosis might originate from the effects of abuse, but also long-term life difficulties, motivations, memories, social history, and struggles to narrate and understand. One chapter focuses on refugees who suffered trauma as adults and later became psychotic. Another chapter examines how trauma leads to the destruction of certainty and trust, thereby opening a pathway to persecutory ideas. Drawing on a developmental model of trauma, it is proposed that dissociated parts of the self that developed during childhood contribute to psychosis in adults when undergoing difficulties and stress.

Presented with case illustrations, the book will be useful for those who work in the area of psychosis and abuse to understand the experiences of individuals, and how we might develop appropriate therapy and care.

John Rhodes is a Consultant Clinical Psychologist and a Visiting Lecturer at the University of Hertfordshire. He wrote *Narrative CBT: Distinctive Features* (2014) and co-authored *Narrative CBT for Psychosis* (2009). He has published articles in the areas of psychosis, trauma, and depression.

PSYCHOSIS AND
THE TRAUMATISED SELF

Understanding and Change

John Rhodes

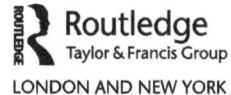
Routledge
Taylor & Francis Group

LONDON AND NEW YORK

Cover image credit: © Getty images

First published 2022
by Routledge
4 Park Square, Milton Park, Abingdon, Oxon OX14 4RN

and by Routledge
605 Third Avenue, New York, NY 10158

Routledge is an imprint of the Taylor & Francis Group, an informa business

© 2022 John Rhodes

British Library Cataloguing-in-Publication Data
A catalogue record for this book is available from the British Library

Library of Congress Cataloging-in-Publication Data
Names: Rhodes, John, author.
Title: Psychosis and the traumatised self : understanding and change / John Rhodes.
Description: Milton Park, Abingdon, Oxon ; New York, NY : Routledge, 2022. | Includes bibliographical references and index. |
Identifiers: LCCN 2021048094 (print) | LCCN 2021048095 (ebook) | ISBN 9780367491864 (hardback) | ISBN 9780367491796 (paperback) | ISBN 9781003044956 (ebook) Subjects: LCSH: Psychoses. | Psychoses--Treatment. | Psychoses in children.
Classification: LCC RC512 .R46 2022 (print) | LCC RC512 (ebook) | DDC 616.89--dc23/eng/20211124
LC record available at https://lccn.loc.gov/2021048094
LC ebook record available at https://lccn.loc.gov/2021048095

ISBN: 978-0-367-49186-4 (hbk)
ISBN: 978-0-367-49179-6 (pbk)
ISBN: 978-1-003-04495-6 (ebk)

DOI: 10.4324/9781003044956

Typeset in Joanna
by MPS Limited, Dehradun

CONTENTS

ACKNOWLEDGEMENTS

I wish to thank Richard Gipps, Natasha Vorontsova, Luke Bosdet, Simon Jakes, Peter Howson, Natan Barreto, Joanna Farr, who have all contributed in many different ways.

I also wish to thank Louise Healey, Nathan O'Neill, Neil Parrett, Pieter Nel, and Oliver Mason for the contributions they made in carrying out the research presented in the book.

Finally, I wish to thank and acknowledge the bravery of the participants who kindly agreed to be interviewed for the research.

1

PSYCHOSIS AND TRAUMA

After just a few years of working with psychosis, two new clients began therapy with me and asked to talk about the abuse and trauma that had occurred in their lives. One had experienced extreme physical abuse in childhood and the other had been in a war as an adult. Of course, I had known about the possibility of abuse and trauma beforehand, but meeting individuals who were motivated to talk through this, and who later said that the therapy had helped, changed my way of understanding and doing therapy. It taught me that some clients were able to explore such issues, could benefit from this, and would not deteriorate or somehow come apart. This book presents research and therapeutic applications which came out of such initial explorations and draws on the growing body of relevant findings and theory. In this chapter, I will discuss types of trauma, the general effects of trauma, and consider the relationship between trauma and psychosis in terms of long-term effects and causation. Finally, I will describe how the research for the various chapters was carried out and give a brief overview of the book.

DOI: 10.4324/9781003044956-1

Types of abuse and trauma

There is a range of types of abuse and trauma: the Child Trauma Questionnaire (Bernstein & Fink, 1998) lists physical abuse, sexual abuse, emotional abuse, physical neglect, and emotional neglect. While the term 'trauma' includes the impacts of abuse, it can also result from a wide range of events such as parental death, loss, becoming ill with physical or mental conditions. Sometimes the word 'adversity' is used to include wider phenomena such as poverty or living in difficult environments.

This book explores the experiences of three groups of individuals experiencing psychosis: those who have suffered sexual abuse or physical abuse in childhood and those impacted by trauma in the context of political violence such as torture or war. The wider range of traumas is not covered. In this section, however, I wish to make some comments on the relevance of two sorts of trauma which have typically also occurred in the lives of the three groups looked at in the book, that is, child emotional abuse and the trauma of the onset of psychosis and hospitalisation.

Child emotional abuse and neglect

Child emotional abuse and neglect (Glaser, 2002) can involve any of the following: parental emotional unavailability, parental negative attributions about a child, developmentally inappropriate interactions, failure to recognise individuality and psychological boundaries, using the child for fulfilment of the parents' psychological needs, and failure to promote the child's social adaptation. It has been consistently found (e.g., Cawson et al., 2000; Mason et al., 2009) that some form of emotional abuse usually accompanies other severe forms of child abuse such as sexual and physical abuse. It was assumed that this would probably be true of those participating in the research reported in this book.

Hospitalisation and the onset of psychosis

The onset of psychosis may in itself be such an extreme and negative event that it constitutes a form of trauma. Hutchins, Rhodes, and Keville (2016) noted a very wide range of powerful emotions including shame and guilt following the trauma of breakdown and hospitalisation. The personal meaning of experiencing a mental health crisis can substantially impact an individual's identity, with long-term consequences. In addition to experiencing the disturbing effects of psychosis, a person is often put under the care of the psychiatric system or hospitalised against their will. It is perhaps not surprising that some patients describe their experiences as incarceration, and the fact they are being detained in hospital adds negative meaning to their already heightened concerns.

A review by Berry et al. (2015) showed high levels of post-traumatic stress disorder (PTSD) resulting from the trauma of psychosis or hospitalisation or both, with prevalence rates for PTSD resulting from these traumas varying from 11% to 67%. They also noted that there was some evidence that the severity of psychosis-related PTSD is influenced by the person's previous trauma history. Inpatient psychiatric experience often features disempowerment, coercion, and the restriction of liberty, which can echo conditions of childhood adversity. Given this finding, it is possible that those who have experienced child abuse might find involuntary treatment particularly distressing.

Lu et al. (2017) carried out qualitative work using semi-structured interviews to examine the experience of sixty-three people on an inpatient psychiatric unit who had experienced either a first or multiple episodes of hospitalisation. The main finding was that both the experience of having psychosis and being hospitalised were potentially traumatic. Some features of psychosis which were found to be traumatic included frightening hallucinations, suicidal thoughts, thoughts about harming others, delusions, and unusual behaviours. The patients reported that the psychosis itself also induced anger, sadness, confusion, anxiety, and numbness. In terms of the actual treatment they experienced, the patients mentioned: being kept in hospital for a long time; forced medication; upsetting side effects; coercive treatments involving the use of restraints; being exposed to aggressive patients; and mistreatment by professionals. It is an extremely vivid and worrying picture but, I believe, will be one recognised by those who have worked on wards. Of course some patients somehow cope better with psychosis and many patients do seek help and find their care helpful. It is certainly the case, however, that some patients have a terrible struggle as they are admitted to hospital, particularly during a first episode; and even the most compassionate care may be involuntary and thus constitute a severe challenge to an individual's sense of autonomy and personhood.

The long-term effects of abuse and trauma

Reviewing the experiences of those who have suffered child abuse and protracted trauma in adult years, Herman (1992) suggested a series of criteria for what she termed 'Complex Post-Traumatic Stress Disorder'. Whether this is a useful specific diagnostic category or not, the list of symptoms is certainly an illuminating overview of the effects of abuse. She states that abuse affects a person's ability to regulate and live with their emotions and involves experiencing extreme negative emotions. There can be effects upon consciousness itself such as amnesia or derealisation and specific features of PTSD such as reliving. It affects the person's perception of the self and is associated with feelings of shame, guilt, and self-blame. Herman noted how a person may feel themselves to be completely different from others. There are changes in relationships such that a person can become isolated, withdrawn, and experiences persistent mistrust. There can be a loss of meaning and a sense of hopelessness and despair. In situations of being held captive (e.g., domestic abuse) there can be alterations in the perception of the perpetrator.

A great deal of research has examined the specific long-term effects of early abuse. A review by Anda et al. (2006) noted that the more childhood adversities a person had suffered, the greater the incidence and severity of negative outcomes. Outcomes included the risk of panic reactions, depressed affect, anxiety, and hallucinations; sleep disturbance, severe obesity, and multiple somatic symptoms; substance use and abuse; smoking, alcoholism; risk of early sexual intercourse, multiple sexual partners, and sexual dissatisfaction; impaired memory of childhood; high perceived stress, difficulty controlling anger, and the risk of perpetrating intimate partner violence. A review by Heim et al. (2010) described a similar picture, noting the long-term prevalence of a range of mood and anxiety disorders, schizophrenia, attachment disorder, eating disorders, and personality disorders. They underlined that childhood trauma also dramatically increases the risk for later substance abuse and suicide attempts.

There is now a growing body of research looking at changes that may occur in terms of the brain and nervous systems of persons who have survived childhood abuse (Van der Kolk, 2014). A review by Teicher and Samson (2016) suggests that not only are these changes long lasting, but that there may be specific changes in the brain according to the type of abuse suffered. The authors concluded that 'structural and functional abnormalities initially attributed to psychiatric illness may be a more direct consequence of abuse'. Some reviews have focused specifically on the effects of physical or sexual abuse, and these are given in chapters two and three. From the many pieces of research we can say with confidence that experiencing abuse in childhood is one of the most destructive things possible in a person's life, and leads to a wide range of psychopathologies and other forms of suffering.

Does childhood abuse lead to psychosis?

A great deal of research has now shown that various forms of childhood abuse are highly prevalent in the histories of those diagnosed with psychosis: a review by Read et al. (2005) suggested that 48% of female participants reported sexual abuse and 48% physical abuse, while 29% of male participants reported sexual abuse and 50% physical abuse. The results of a meta-study examining the relation between psychosis and childhood abuse (Varese et al., 2012) suggested that those who had suffered childhood adversity were 2.8 times more likely to have psychosis than those who had not. Matheson et al. (2013) in their meta-study reached the same conclusions. Read and colleagues (Read et al., 2005; Skehan, Larkin & Read, 2012) have argued that such evidence points to the probable causal role of abuse.

Longden et al. (2016) added to the evidence for a causal effect of abuse by demonstrating a dose-response relationship between childhood adversities and psychotic symptoms. They used randomly selected records from New Zealand community mental health centres and found that the higher the number of childhood adversities in a patient's history, the higher the number of psychotic symptoms they later experienced, including hallucinations, delusions, and negative symptoms. Longden and colleagues did not find evidence for specific links of sexual abuse with hallucinations or physical abuse with delusions, although these had been suggested in previous reports. The data were consistent with a model of global and cumulative adversity, in which multiple exposures may intensify the risk of psychosis beyond the impact of single events.

Social and psychological features of those with psychosis and abuse histories

What social or psychological features might be commonly found in adults who have suffered childhood abuse and who have a diagnosis of psychosis? In terms of social problems, Skehan et al. (2012) pointed to higher levels of homelessness, impaired intimacy, and extensive use of psychiatric services. These patients were also more likely to have attempted suicide than patients with psychosis who had not been abused. A recent meta-analysis of features by Rodriguez et al. (2021) noted a wide range of cognitive alterations in working memory, attention, social cognitive processes, and emotional perception.

As well as mapping the psychological profiles of those with psychosis and a history of abuse, research has tried to identify specific features which might perpetuate a person's difficulties, and potentially even constitute causal pathways between childhood trauma and psychosis. Such features have included: 1) post-traumatic sequelae including dissociation, 2) affective dysfunction and dysregulation, and 3) maladaptive cognitive factors such as negative beliefs about self and others. Williams et al. (2018) in a meta-study found evidence for all three of these features mediating the trauma-psychosis link. Another meta-study by Alameda et al. (2020) has in general confirmed the findings of Williams et al., demonstrating particularly solid evidence concerning pathways from childhood abuse to psychosis via post-traumatic symptoms including dissociation, and via negative cognitive schemas about the self, the world, and others.

Isvoranu 2016 et al. (2016) examined evidence for an affective pathway using statistical network analysis (i.e., where any possible relation between all specific symptoms and a very wide range of outcomes is investigated and the strength of statistical association is given). The most common pathway between childhood trauma and all types of later psychotic symptoms was shown to be the experience of anxiety; that is to say that many different types of abuse led to anxiety, and anxiety in its turn was associated with all psychotic symptoms. Two lesser additional pathways indicated by the analysis were via poor impulse control (which connected to areas such as grandiosity and excitement or hostility) and via motor retardation in adults, following neglect in childhood, and leading to later negative symptoms.

Explanatory models

All of the above findings in different ways, and to different degrees, may contribute to the building of causal models, that is, an explanation of how abuse actually leads to psychosis. Several causal or explanatory theories have been suggested; I will not give here detailed accounts but simply highlight some well-known models. Read and colleagues (2014) have explored potential long-term changes in neurological functioning and the central nervous system: their work suggests that trauma in children leads to lasting changes; in particular, they note over-reactivity to stress of the hypothalamic–pituitary–adrenal axis and the dopaminergic system. They also note changes in the hippocampus and frontal lobes. They argue that the changes formed by abuse lead to the same sorts of cognitive deficit found in participants with psychosis.

Cognitive models have emphasised the importance of meaning and interpretation of experiences. Morrison et al. (2003) argued that those experiencing psychosis, as well as those with trauma history, suffer from 'intrusive' experiences (e.g., thoughts, memories, impulses), and that in psychosis these intrusions are interpreted in culturally unacceptable ways; a person might believe that an intrusive thought relating to past trauma has been inserted by an external agent, rather than coming from a part of their own mind. Steel et al. (2005) argued that 'contextual integration' is a central feature in understanding trauma and psychosis; it is noted that a traumatic experience might be so overwhelming that normal memory processes are interrupted such that instead of remembering a terrible image as something from the distant past, it may be experienced as occurring in the present moment. This triggers a search for meaning; the person may imagine, for example, that they are under attack or surveillance by a gang.

Hardy (2017) has developed a model that includes an interaction of memory processes, dissociation, emotional dysregulation, self and other cognitions, and appraisal of intrusions and their consequences. In brief, emotional dysregulation makes it more likely that intrusive experiences associated with memory disruption and dissociation are triggered, negative cognitive structures make it more likely that these are interpreted in a threatening way, and the combination of these with avoidant coping strategies can prevent reprocessing of memories and reappraisal of beliefs.

Dissociation is a concept with an extensive history as a core process in trauma and psychosis (Ross, 2004; Van der Hart, Niejenhuis & Steele, 2006; Moskowitz, Dorahy, Schäfer, 2019). Dissociation has been conceptualised in many ways, from subjectively experienced states of depersonalisation and derealisation, through to 'structural dissociation', that is, a state whereby mental processes that normally cohere, interconnect, and function together are to various degrees rendered separate and can in extreme cases involve an apparent fragmentation of the personality. I will return to this concept in later chapters.

Given the multitude of diverse findings and theories, it might be that eventually all these different ways of describing and explaining the phenomena could be fused into a multilevel integrative model and one that includes social events, meaning, social processes, psychological processes, and neurological change. I believe it will also need to include findings from the first person perspective, qualitative research, and phenomenology.

Research presented in this book

Clearly trauma is an extremely important issue concerning those who experience psychosis, and that is the case whether we consider it primarily as a causal factor or as an additional burden. In the literature it has been suggested there are several pathways to psychosis, some being initiated by biological events and others from trauma. It is possible that for some patients they suffered both biological causes and abuse simultaneously. Whatever the pathway, it is important that we understand the nature of the experience. Earlier in the chapter I presented quantitative research which maps not only potential causes and effects but the actual features and processes which may be contributing to the development of psychosis. However, all of these quantitative pieces of research cannot describe what participants perceive as occurring or important, or the experience of everyday life in its complexity, or how for an individual the different features may interact or amplify each other.

In addition to understanding abuse in general it is also important that we understand the possible effects of specific types of trauma; for example, are the long-term consequences suffered by participants who survived sexual abuse different from those who have experienced physical abuse? Furthermore, what are the immediate experiences of those who have undergone terrible traumas during adult years such as domestic violence or war? Are those who suffer trauma in their adult years affected differently from those who experience abuse in childhood?

The importance of understanding the actual experience of participants in its complexity led to the various pieces of research upon which this book draws and expands. In the first part of the book three separate but coordinated pieces of research carried out by myself and colleagues are reported in detail: chapter one looks at child physical abuse, chapter two at child sexual abuse, and chapter three at refugees who have suffered forms of political violence. For these pieces of research a deliberate effort was made to find participants who had suffered only physical abuse or only sexual abuse and not several types of child abuse simultaneously (except of course emotional abuse, which we assumed would also be present as described earlier). We hoped that by investigating the different types of abuse separately, we would have more confidence in any findings concerning the different effects and experiences.

For the research we used a methodology called interpretive phenomenological analysis (IPA), developed by Smith and colleagues (Smith et al., 2009). The approach involves interviewing in depth a small number of participants. A central aim of this methodology is to capture a participant's experience of a phenomenon and the meaning it holds for them. While it is concerned with personal experience, IPA's primary focus is those experiences that are important to people and prompt reflection. The method is interpretive or 'hermeneutical' in that it assumes that meaning is central to experience and that the meaning of an experience for a person only comes to light, and can be seen, through the interpretative process. The approach draws from phenomenology, in that it tries to capture the world and self as experienced, as it appears, and not as it might be assumed in a psychological or other theory. While phenomenology emphasises the immediate experience of the person, it also sees the person and their experiences as immersed in a practical, historical, and cultural context and inseparable from it. In fact, the tradition of phenomenology asks us to think of persons as existing in concrete and cultural contexts and that individuals and social contexts co-created each other. IPA, however, is a psychological method and is not a way of doing a type of philosophy. After the initial analysis of findings, and the generation of themes, it aims to stay close to a person's experience and rooted in the data; quite often IPA then relates findings to ideas in psychology or social sciences and might also draw, if appropriate, upon ideas from phenomenology and other philosophies during extended conceptual analysis. I would argue that IPA does not rely upon phenomenology as a 'method' but rather as a conceptual framework or as a 'topic' area, the latter being the lived world, the self, the other, and context as manifest and given in experience.

IPA was also used because it is idiographic, focuses on experience, has a well worked out set of procedures that specify how the interview should be structured, and how the interviews can be analysed. It specifies how each case is analysed ideographically, and a table of themes is established before moving to the next case. A cross case analysis of the table of themes from each participant is conducted to create a superordinate table of themes for all participants in the study.

The themes may occur at different levels, for example, quite specific themes or more general themes which capture variations. The process is, however, complex, and involves discussion, comparison, and further thought and often new cycles of analysis until a coherent set of ideas is generated. The themes generated from the three groups are presented in chapters two, three, and four. This book, however, also involves further extended analysis. In chapters five, six, and seven there are comparisons made between the three groups and explicit links are made to a range of psychological and sometimes phenomenological concepts and theories.

The participants

The three groups were interviewed with a similar set of questions (though with some altered details for each group). The questions were about the participants present lives, their experiences over the years, what difficulties and problems they were suffering from, and issues such as 'voices' if these were mentioned in the interview. There was also a focus on how they saw the effects of abuse over their lives. We did not, however, focus on details of the abuse itself which we thought would be not necessary for this research and might be disturbing for the participant. We aimed not to introduce psychiatric language into the interviews, but did find that many participants would spontaneously use terms such as 'voices' or 'paranoid' which allowed discussion of these features.

To find possible participants we relied on information in notes and reports from psychiatrists and psychologists based in a community psychiatric service and hospital. Trauma histories were assessed using the Child Trauma Questionnaire (Bernstein & Fink, 1998), which has been used in many pieces of research with trauma and psychosis. The questionnaire is succinct and does not go into disturbing detail.

For the study of refugee experiences, we sought asylum seekers who had reported histories of exposure to violence in their countries of origin and had displayed psychotic symptoms, as recorded by psychiatrists, while in the UK. Permission to carry out the research was given by the local ethics committee. All potential participants were given a full explanation of the project and choice as to whether to participate. Furthermore, if participants were not happy about the interview they were able to request that the data would be erased (no one requested this).

Outline of the book

After the introductory chapter the book has three main parts. In the chapters two to four, detailed findings are presented from research with participants who suffered sexual or physical abuse in childhood or suffered in the context of political violence and became refugees. In chapters five to seven, comparisons will be made across the three groups and further analysis on key topics is given. In chapter five it will be argued that psychotic meanings found in voices and delusions, but also in everyday social perceptions, relate to specific past traumas. There is also a review of the many contributions to delusional meanings and a full case study. Chapter six presents evidence describing extreme emotional and interpersonal states and how these may be transformed in psychosis: this is also linked to the perception of others and voices. In chapter seven it is argued that psychosis involves the disturbance of a person's grasp of the shared everyday world, of basic certainties and trust, and that these are influenced by trauma. Finally, there is a focus on therapy; in chapter eight models of therapy suitable for work with trauma and psychosis are discussed and ideas for modifying schema therapy given. Chapter nine contains detailed examples of such work and an extended case illustration.

References

Alameda, L., Rodriguez, V., Carr, E., Aas, M., Trotta, G., Marino, P., ... Murray, R.M. (2020). A systematic review on mediators between adversity and psychosis: Potential targets for treatment. *Psychological Medicine, 50,* 1966–1976.

Anda, R., Felitti, V., Bremner, J., Walker, J., Whitfield, C., Perry, B., ... Giles, W.H. (2006). The enduring effects of abuse and related adverse experiences in childhood. *European Archives of Psychiatry and Clinical Neuroscience, 256,* 174–186.

Bernstein, D.P., & Fink, L. (1998). *Childhood trauma questionnaire: A retrospective self-report manual.* San Antonio, TX: Psychological Corporation.

Berry, K., Ford, S., Jellicoe-Jones, L., & Haddock, G. (2015). Trauma in relation to psychosis and hospital experiences: The role of past trauma and attachment. *Psychology and Psychotherapy: Theory, Research and Practice, 88,* 227–239.

Cawson, P., Wattam, C., Brooker, S., & Kelly, G. (2000). *Child Maltreatment in the United Kingdom: A study of the prevalence of child abuse and neglect.* London: NSPCC.

Glaser, D. (2002). Emotional abuse and neglect (psychological maltreatment): A conceptual framework. *Child Abuse and Neglect, 26,* 697–714.

Hardy, A. (2017). Pathways from trauma to psychotic experiences: A theoretically informed model of posttraumatic stress in psychosis. *Frontiers in Psychology, 8,* 697–717.

Herman, J.L. (1992). *Trauma and recovery.* New York: Basic Books.

Heim, C., Shugart, M., Craighead, W.E., & Nemeroff, C.B. (2010). Neurobiological and psychiatric consequences of child abuse and neglect. *Developmental Psychobiology, 52,* 671–690.

Hutchins, J., Rhodes, J., & Keville, S. (2016). Emotional earthquakes in the landscape of psychosis: an interpretative phenomenology. *The Cognitive Behaviour Therapist, 9,* e30. doi: 10.1017/S1754470X16000167.

Isvoranu, A.-M., van Borkulo, C.D., Boyette, L.L., Wigman, J.T.W., Vinkers, C.H., & Borsboom, D. (2016). A network approach to psychosis: pathways between childhood trauma and psychotic symptoms. *Schizophrenia Bulletin, 43,* 187–196.

Longden, E., Sampson, M., & Read, J. (2015). Childhood adversity and psychosis: Generalised or specific effects? *Epidemiology and Psychiatric Sciences, 25,* 349–359.

Lu, W., Mueser, K.T., Rosenberg, S.D., Yanos, P.T., & Mahmoud, N. (2017). Posttraumatic reactions to psychosis: A qualitative analysis. *Frontiers in Psychiatry*, *8*, 129. 10.3389/fpsyt.2017.00129.

Matheson, S.L., Shepherd, A.M., Pinchbeck, R.M., Laurns, K.R., & Carr, V.J. (2013). Childhood adversity in schizophrenia: A systematic meta-analysis. *Psychological Medicine*, *43*, 225–238.

Mason, O., Brett, E., Collinge, M., Curr, H., & Rhodes J. (2009). Child abuse and the content of delusions. *Child Abuse and Neglect*, *33*(4), 205–208.

Morrison, A.P., Frame, L., & Larkin, W. (2003). Relationships between trauma and psychosis: A review and integration. *British Journal of Clinical Psychology*, *42*, 331–353.

Moskowitz, A., Dorahy, M.J., & Schäfer, I. (2019). *Psychosis, Trauma and Dissociation: Evolving Perspectives on Severe Psychopathology*, (2nd ed.), London: Wiley.

Read, J., Fosse, R., Moskowitz, A., & Perry, B. (2014). The traumagenic neurodevelopmental model of psychosis revisited. *Neuropsychiatry*, *4*, 65–79.

Read, J., van Os, J., Morrison, A.P., & Ross, C.A. (2005). Childhood trauma, psychosis and schizophrenia: A literature review with theoretical and clinical implications. *Acta Psychiatrica Scandinavica*, *112*, 330–350.

Rodriguez, V., Aas, M., Vorontsova, N., Trotta, G., Gadelrab, R., Rooprai, N.K., & Alameda, L. (2021). Exploring the interplay between adversity, neurocognition, social cognition, and functional outcome in people with psychosis: A narrative review. *Frontiers in Psychiatry*, *12*: doi: 10.3389/fpsyt.2 021.596949.

Ross, C.A. (2004). *Schizophrenia: Innovations in diagnosis and treatment*. New York, NY: Haworth Press.

Skehan, D., Larkin, Q., & Read, J. (2012). Childhood adversity and psychosis: A literature review with clinical and societal implications. *Psychoanalysis, Culture & Society*, *17*, 373–391.

Smith, J.A., Flowers, P., & Larkin, M. (2009). *Interpretative Phenomenological Analysis: Theory, Method, and Research*. London: Sage.

Steel, C., Fowler, D., & Holmes, E.A. (2005). Trama-related intrusions and psychosis: An information processing account. *Behavioural and Cognitive Psychotherapy*, *33*, 139–152.

Teicher, M.H., & Samson, J.A. (2016). Annual research review: Enduring neurobiological effects of childhood abuse and neglect. *Journal of Child Psychology and Psychiatry*, *57*, 241–266.

Van der Kolk, B.A. (2014). *The body keeps the score: brain, mind and body in the healing of trauma*. New York: Viking Press.

Van der Hart, O., Niejenhuis, E., & Steele, K. (2006). *The haunted self: Structural dissociation and the treatment of chronic traumatisation*. New York, USA: Norton.

Varese, F., Smeets, F., Drukker, M., Lieverse, R., Lataster, T., Viechbauer, ... Bentall, R.P. (2012). Childhood adversities increase the risk of psychosis: a meta-analysis of patient-control, prospective- and cross-sectional cohort studies. *Schizophrenia Bulletin, 38*, 661–671.

Williams, J., Bucci, S., Berry, K., & Varese, F. (2018). Psychological mediators of the association between childhood adversities and psychosis: A systematic review. *Clinical Psychology Review, 65*, 175–196.

2

PHYSICAL ABUSE AND PSYCHOSIS

Introduction

Physical abuse is a terrible and harmful assault on the person, and may cause or contribute to psychosis. The focus of this chapter is to present first person experiential reports of adults diagnosed with psychosis and who underwent physical abuse in childhood. In short, what has their experience been like over recent years, what are their concerns? The chapter is a revised version of Rhodes and Healey (2016).[1] First, however, I will briefly present some specific research findings connecting child physical abuse (CPA) with psychosis.

The long term consequences of child physical abuse

Several studies have mapped out the long-term consequences of experiencing CPA. In research by Springer et al. (2007) looking at data from 2,800 adults in the general population, the results suggested that 11.4% reported CPA; those with physical abuse were found to have high levels of

DOI: 10.4324/9781003044956-2

depression, anxiety, anger, physical symptoms, and medical diagnoses. In another community survey (Sugaya et al., 2012) looking at 43,093 participants, 8% were found to report CPA; controlling for other variables the research suggested that there is an increased chance among those with physical abuse of going on to experience attention deficit hyperactivity disorder, post-traumatic stress disorder, and bipolar disorder. They also noticed that there was a 'dose-response effect', that is, the more abuse experienced, the more likely one would be to be diagnosed with these conditions. Clearly the effects of CPA are powerful and destructive in the lives of adults.

Child physical abuse and adult survivors with psychosis

Chapter one summarised the research looking at a range of types of childhood abuse and included the potential link between physical abuse with later psychosis. Fisher et al. (2014) reported a specific association between CPA and psychotic symptoms; furthermore, their analysis suggested that this association was independent of family psychiatric history, that is, they were able to account for the possible genetic influence of parents and to still show that CPA was an independent predictor of later psychosis.

Bullying

The focus of this chapter is not on bullying, which is conceived as being carried out by a person's peer group outside the family, and is not usually classified as CPA. However, it is clear that the two involve similar elements of physical violence and intimidation. It is therefore interesting to note that research (Cunningham et al., 2016) has suggested that bullying itself may be another influence on a pathway to psychosis, particularly late onset psychosis.

The participants

All the participants for this research scored highly on the Childhood Trauma Questionnaire (CTQ; Bernstein & Fink, 1998). The CTQ defines

CPA as 'bodily assaults on a child by an older person that pose a risk of, or result in, injury'. This is the definition we assumed for this book. Eight adult participants experiencing psychosis were recruited from a psychiatric facility in London. Diagnoses were identified from clinical records. As is recommended in interpretive phenomenological analysis (IPA), we aimed to recruit a small number of participants, and those recruited were the first eight to meet our criteria. Participant details and abuse histories are shown in Table 2.1.

The participants were asked when the physical abuse that they experienced began and ended, the frequency, and who carried out the abuse. In sum, the abuse was mainly classified on the CTQ as 'severe to extreme'; the abuse had been carried out by one or both parents, often started below the age of eight, and ended during the person's late teens. The abuse occurred regularly, often on a weekly basis. The participants had no documented experiences of childhood sexual abuse and did not score for sexual abuse on the CTQ.

The themes expressed by participants

The following themes were generated: aggression-permeated world; de-humanising self attack; pervasive mistrust and the 'front' of others; damaged intimacy; the fluctuating 'thread' of meaning and identity

Table 2.1 Characteristics of participants

Participants	Age (years)	Gender	Ethnicity	Diagnoses
Mirza	53	M	Asian British	Schizoaffective disorder
Peter	42	M	White British	Bipolar disorder with psychotic features
Chris	34	M	Nigerian British	Paranoid schizophrenia
Lesley	23	F	White Irish	Paranoid schizophrenia
William	48	M	White Irish	Paranoid schizophrenia
Greg	32	M	Black Mixed Heritage British	Drug-induced psychotic episodes
Sally	32	F	White British	Schizoaffective disorder
Rita	38	F	Black British	Paranoid schizophrenia

transformations; dread of murderous obliteration; distress and perceived links to the past.

Aggression-permeated world

All the participants saw other people in general as difficult and often dangerous. The other might actually attack physically, but short of that, is seen as emanating hate, rejection, and sometimes contempt. Mirza said:

> I've been mugged and beaten up quite a lot walking the streets, you know? Sometimes I feel scared to go out ... Well you're just ... locked up in a prison, you know? And you feel locked up, umm, even though you've got your freedom you know? You can go out that door anytime you want to, you don't, you're scared to go out that door.

He states that he is in danger and that someone will attack him: further, this is how things are every day. It is not just a possibility, but an actual threat. The door seems a slender barrier. He went on to say:

> You see people abusing each other in the papers. People are generally that way ... life's not a bed of roses ... many people die in the hurricane.

To be alive is to experience a hurricane: it is to be exposed to a huge uncontrollable violent force. While the rose image is well known, perhaps a cliché, the next phrase conveys both sadness and fear. All one can do is try to shelter and hide, but then one is a prisoner. In the hurricane,

> Many don't get to see the end of their lives.

They do not see what is supposed to be the natural end, but rather, what they see is their own untimely violent death. Mirza's hurricane, however, is not one of nature, it is other people and what they are willing to do. For some participants, the zone of threat is more specific:

> You'll follow a certain crowd and you end up in certain parts of society, and in those certain parts it's, that's the only thing that goes on, fights, stabbings, shootings and all that. (Chris)

The world he lives in is one of violence; it is the norm, the 'only' thing. With a similar emphasis on violence, Sally stated about her ex-partner:

He would go off big time. He'd start throwing me about, getting nasty.

This partner of seven years was not only violent but 'nasty', suggesting he did this not just as a sudden explosion of emotion, but with deliberate hostile intention. The reported world of the participants was one of extreme fear of violence. Whether this was just what might be thought of as a misperception, or that in fact they did live in social worlds with more violence, cannot be answered here.

Dehumanising self attack

Six participants spontaneously described negative attitudes to themselves: two were almost violent in their self attack. Greg stated:

Always looking and seeing myself as ugly and fat and unattractive... it's just like 'there's a pin, there's another pin' like a voodoo doll, 'there's another pin'.

He represents himself as a 'voodoo doll' which he torments with pins. A 'doll' is usually childlike and here it is as if he attacks some part of himself that is childlike. A voodoo doll is used to hurt someone: the person in this case appears to be Greg himself. In this one complex blended image he expresses attacking and being attacked within himself.

William also described 'self attack':

Running myself down, you know, saying you're a fool, you're an idiot, you're, very nasty things to myself ... your brain is screwed, you're never going to be right in the head.

The image seems very much one of one person shouting at another an endless stream of insults. In the above, William speaks in the second person, as if in a dialogue. He seems to be speaking in the voice of one who is superior and aggressive to one who is silent and inferior, who just takes this stream of attack. It is reminiscent of someone authoritarian and of 'telling off'.

While six participants directly held negative views of themselves (from extreme to moderate), of these six a further four also expressed the idea that others saw them in negative ways. While Sally felt that she was 'disgusting and dirty' she also noted how difficult her relationship was with her son,

> I feel he's not knowing me as me, he's knowing some monster ...

Her son not only perceives her apparent state as monstrous, but he 'knows', suggesting a deeper knowledge perhaps developed over many encounters. But what is a monster? Perhaps something that is destructive and not even human. Further, if he 'knows' he is unlikely to change his view easily. The statement suggests a sense of pessimism.

In contrast to several others, Peter did not criticise himself, but was tormented by how others saw him and in particular, a neighbour:

> They see a monster. Each day she turns me into a monster ... I seem to be wearing this big sandwich board saying 'freak, pervert', and whatever, you know.

That she is able to turn him into a monster seems to suggest not only that she sees him in that way, but that she contributes to this process doing it bit by bit each day. It is interesting to note how two participants used the actual word 'monster'.

Pervasive mistrust and the 'front' of others

Six participants expressed a sense of extreme mistrust, either directly or indirectly. While mistrust and the theme of a hostile world were often found in combination, it was clear that mistrust and confusion extended to many other contexts. Lesley stated:

> I don't really know when a friend's a friend.

For most of us this is not a problem, we know our friends and continue to feel confident even during arguments. But Lesley does not know: she is cut off from whatever it is that creates trust. Sally claimed that a social worker (in fact there for her child) had begun a relation with her boyfriend: ' ... and I felt her going off in the car with him'.

It is interesting to note how she says 'felt', that is, not something seen or heard. She has a feeling of the person actually going off with another. The 'going off' appears to be both spatial and social. Her mistrust is much deeper than a mere guess or idea. Peter also does not believe the appearance of everyday events and interactions: ' ... being able to quite often see through lies and mistruths, through people's body language, through their, just general vibe'.

What is presented by the other is not believed. He says the above as if it were a general truth of his social world. There is something to 'see through', that is, what is said and how others behave, and this surface must conceal the truth. The experience of the everyday world as having some sort of surface that conceals was conspicuous for Mirza:

> They are just putting on a front ... inside they want to kill you, they want to murder you, they want to do bad things to you.

In the world of Mirza, there remains, despite appearances, the likelihood that others hide murderous intentions. In the everyday world, we assume, more or less, that the friendliness we see in others is just that. His world seems a lonely and fearful one: it contains Mirza, the 'front' of others, and their unknown but suspected malicious intentions. The behaviour of others has no intrinsic meaning or worth: it is just a surface that conceals.

Damaged intimacy

This theme concerns damaged intimacy, that is, the person's profound difficulty in maintaining good relationships with partners or friends, and with it a sense of loneliness. All the participants reported difficulties with intimate relationships, and few were in relationships. While four explicitly mentioned anger or aggression by the other affecting their relationships (see Sally in the theme of hostility), four thought others saw them as angry, and of these, two were sure of their own repeated extreme anger at others. Rita spoke openly of being:

> Verbally abusive, umm, emotionally abusive ... I tremble and shake with temper.

She is out of control and appears transformed. The body 'shakes' as if some force had overwhelmed her. Over time she found herself in the situation of being: …

very, very lonely and isolated.

In all, six participants described intimacy difficulties involving hostility from self or from the other. William described feeling great anger at others (which he hid) but was also very aware of his isolation and disconnection from others:

I've never really, I've never really been truly involved with people, you know, on an emotional level.

He added that throughout his life he had been:

Incapable of the emotions, of the deep emotion, or I've been unwilling to involve myself with it.

He knows there is such a thing as 'deep emotion', yet is not able to have this experience. He qualifies his statement by adding that he might have been 'unwilling' to be involved, as though he sometimes blamed himself, as if this was somehow voluntary. Irrespective of blame, his predicament suggests the most profound long-term loneliness. It is to live in a world where one is alone and interaction is only superficial and distant. And in a sense, he performs this lack of involvement in the apparent calm of coolly presenting his statements as being either/or, as if making a legal or scientific argument.

Peter reported feeling no anger at others but stated that others feared him and did not understand him. In the following Peter describes profound loneliness:

People's misconceptions of me, their misunderstanding, their inability to be able to talk to me, … That hurts the most, that has the largest impact on my life … I do need communication like all human beings need on occasion. And if I'm starved of that, then it hurts and I start frowning and they think I'm angry, so now I've gotta smile, but the smile, a false smile, yeah with the hope that someone will say 'hello'.

This paints a picture of someone not with others, not understood, and struggling to know how to cope in loneliness that hurts. He does not even receive 'communication', something we mostly take for granted. He resorts to a 'false' smile to have any interaction at all. To understand this position, we need to image a situation where we are left just hoping for a 'hello' from anyone at all.

Paranoia, the fluctuating 'thread' of meaning and identity transformation

Six participants explicitly described the process of what they called 'paranoia', and five in particular described how this process varied over time such that there were moments of strong conviction (e.g., in a plot) but for the rest of time, the ideas and conviction varied. The latter participants positioned themselves at present as not being under the sway of these ideas and feelings; however, it was clear that sometimes they were prone to succumb to what appears to be a sort of force. Often there was fluctuating suspicion and fear. William stated:

> I'm still inclined to visit the paranoia ... there's still a thread in my head ... It sort of develops, usually over a couple of days and then I have a serious, umm, attack if you like, and then it dissipates over a few days.

A thread, involving both meaning and feelings, persists over time and mutates in moments of increased distress. When the 'thread' becomes strong:

> It's unpleasant and very debilitating ... it all seems to fit and it all makes sense ... I've lost the confidence if you like of just normal thought or having a thought and you know, it goes in and out of your head and that's the end of it ... they hang about in the wrong context, in ... feelings of bad luck, or you know, bad experiences ... they're related to a depressive state, where I become depressed to a certain level.

The 'right context' appears to be one of feeling good and being able to dismiss these things with confidence, something we usually take for granted. The 'wrong context' may well be moments of suffering, of a depressive state, and of experiencing memories of 'bad luck'. The latter term seems a way of distancing himself from what was in fact terrible abuse and mistreatment. Concerning the content of his ideas he added:

> I'm still inclined to see it there ... because I was seen as a specimen for manipulation.

The thread is the mutating narrative that he has been a target of experimentation, and that, in fact, he had been placed with abusive foster carers to find out something, to spy, and that this had continued into his adult life. The thread may change over time, but strands of meaning are often repeated. We can perhaps extend William's metaphor by imagining that sometimes the thread is thin, but then is woven until thick, embroiling the person's mind in multiple strands, causing confusion and obscuring his sight.

Lesley described paranoia as a 'bubbling hot pot in my head' suggesting some sort of force or heat, and something bursting out into her mind or experience. And Chris mentioned: 'a feeling of compulsion … they're very, overwhelming', but also a 'feeling of persecution'. And when it occurs:

> I have a panicky sensation in my body … I feel like my body temperature's rising or, umm, I'm too aware of people's reaction and stuff like that.

All the above suggests the forcefulness of the experience, that there is more than 'thinking', but powerful feelings, and ones involving the body. Greg noted how some of his thoughts were not 'normal', but like a 'compulsion'. He states: ' … sort of like a satellite, picking up signals but the signals that you're picking you're distorting and manipulating and bringing them back to you'.

Like William, he noted the repetition of ideas over time:

> And like the paedophile thing was when I first fell ill and I thought I'd done the killings so this all relates back to the very first paranoia experience, which was the most traumatic. And different events I've been paranoid about, I've attached it and it's attached itself, each time I fall ill the same, umm the same, umm, symptoms from one of them, carry on to the next time I fall ill and it breaks down.

The 'satellite' picks up information, warps it, and in doing so, 'attaches' the worst idea of himself to events (and perhaps events to the idea). Over time, similar paranoid ideas 'carry on' to the next episode of breakdown. Greg also described details concerning the actual experience:

> It's like a sort of torture, but thriving off it … and putting yourself down by these thoughts … you know it's, nothing you, nothing to do with you in that sense, but it's just this compulsion to draw in and you know poke the fire and keep it burning.

It is torture yet there is a compulsion to do it, and the process continues. Greg underlined how unpleasant this process is by a contrast with times he is without these ideas and feelings:

> I feel like I'm living, I'm actually living. That's what it feels like, and it feels like there is life, feels like a different person. It's like you haven't got this weight of, of, of these paranoid thoughts weighting down on you, taking, consuming so much of your time.

Here Greg indicates that the paranoia involves a radical transformation of the self, that he is not the same person when unwell. Five participants mentioned alterations in what might be thought of as a sense of 'identity' or self. Two in the midst of breakdown thought they had become children. Peter stated:

> I remembered kneeling in front of … she's full of feeling, full of care … I was at this particular point, I was a child and I went up to her and knelt.

And Lesley:

> I just got very scared of death, I got so sort of like quiet, I turned into like a little girl sort of like, I don't know, I can't describe it.

In contrast, Greg stated, 'I became Jupiter' suggesting something very powerful. Chris while feeling fear and persecution began to think he was a disciple:

> I thought to myself, if I'm feeling this, like this I must be somebody like one of the disciples that's reincarnated and that's why I'm under this feeling of persecution.

It seems that transformation of experienced identity can occur in very different contexts, and ones involving powerful emotions and thoughts.

The 'paranoid' process appears to involve extreme negative claims about what is going on, but in the 'context' of feelings of compulsion, where ideas make clear and persuasive sense. It is as if the experience of the ideas themselves is different, that they have a sort of compelling draw. For some participants at extreme moments during such processes they come to believe and experience themselves as actually having a new identity.

The dread of murderous obliteration

Several discussed either hearing voices or seeing things: in contrast to paranoia, the source of the voices for the participants tended to be less clear. Some participants thought they were related to not being well, but for others they were understood to be coming from the external world. For some participants their source appeared to waver between the two. While there was a great range of ideas expressed as themes in paranoia or voices, one of the most common and vivid was the theme of extreme violence in different forms. Seven participants experienced either voices or visions. Two with voices said:

> They said they were coming to kill me. (Rita)

> I could hear ... 'oh, I'm going to kill you'. (Greg)

The participants are living in a situation where they hear someone wants to kill them and wants to do this on purpose. In states of paranoia, several also had experiences involving the threat of violence or the idea of killing. Here is a selection:

> I see these people as plotting against me, are ready to kill me. (William) ... either kill me, put me in prison, or slowly manipulating my mind'. (Greg)

The attacking entities wish to torture and murder. Lesley in yet more extreme visions reported:

> My back felt like it had been ripped open and I could see all these demons in the mirror and I was screaming and screaming and screaming,

and at another time she also had ideas of being destroyed:

> I suddenly thought I'm going to be killed ... I thought I was going to be cut up into lots of tiny pieces.

Here she is completely obliterated. Not just killed and left at that, but cut into 'tiny pieces'. What entity would do that? What does she fear? One can only imagine something monstrous and cruel, which wants to destroy any trace of her existence.

Distress and perceived links to the past

Having depression and extremely negative emotions was common among the participants: six of the participants had a combination of depression, fear, and feelings of anger. All of the participants expressed aspects of anxiety, and of these, seven were also depressed. When asked to describe her depression, Lesley stated:

> I tried to commit suicide earlier on last year, and I got a really low point a couple of nights ago. I sent my friend a text saying ' ... life's screwing me tight and every positive influence is being taken away from me ... ' I get like that sometimes; umm and I start thinking about all the negative things ... It's got easier to deal with recently, but before I had myself going round in circles biting my jaw or something, thinking everyone could hear what I was thinking.

She not only suffers depression and suicidal thinking, but has an experience of others hearing her thoughts. She is involved in a terrible tangle of feelings and actions.

Often the participants made links between their suffering and the past. Mirza concerning anger stated:

> Well thinking about them, when you think about them then they can make you wanna get vengeance, you know?

Chris also described a form of fear linked to his being abused:

I: Is that what it was like as a child?

R: Yeah, yeah as soon as I hear her footsteps I thought, 'Oh no I'm going to get a beating now', it was like that.

I: And how did you feel?

R: I had panicky feeling and now looking back I think I developed all that, from then.

Rita described several very negative experiences:

Very low, very depressed and sometimes I get very depressed with the voices and also, just about my life, because I've been through so much that you know? In my life, that it sometimes gets me down.

She also experienced anxiety and made direct links to the past:

I was always very frightened; always afraid because of that I had quite a bit of anxiety. I mean I've had anxiety as an adult and I traced it back to then. It was always the anxiety of 'oh, is she coming? What mood will she be in? Will she lash out'? That was anxiety so I knew what anxiety was. It started when I was very, very young.

However, concerning voices Rita stated:

I think it's a possibility but I can't say for definite, it might have done, yes. But I don't see how what I went through as a child could bring on voices. But the mental distress I can understand, but the voices, no.

As stated, all saw some connection between child abuse and their adult suffering. It is interesting to note that, in contrast to the clear link of past events and adult negative emotions, only two (William and Lesley) of the participants stated that they thought their psychotic experience was somehow a product of their childhood. All the others either gave uncertain responses or clearly stated that they saw no connection.

Overview of interview themes

The participants described a lived world of threat, danger, potential violence, and contempt. The other could do terrible things, even when appearances suggested otherwise. They saw themselves as isolated, not connected to others, and prone to deep mistrust. The actual content of paranoia and reported voices quite often suggested the fear of not only being killed but obliterated. The world is a dangerous, terrible, and hopeless place, expressed dramatically by the phrase, 'many die in the hurricane'. All expressed fear, and most reported depression and feelings of anger: the participants saw these as connected to their early experience, but usually did not see voices or paranoia in a similar way. Six of the eight participants explicitly described experiences they saw as 'paranoid', and for some this process seemed compulsive and fluctuating over time. These experiences seem to be periods when their paranoid experiences intensified and were all pervasive. Sometimes during such periods there appeared to be a change in identity, such as experiencing oneself as a child.

Periods of extreme paranoia were described as a radical experiential transformation: it was a process that seemed to overwhelm participants who felt a sort of compulsion, and who found this process painful and disturbing. For those who fluctuated in and out of extreme 'paranoia', the state is clearly not just one of having ideas about persecution and, say, an emotion such as fear. Rather, it seemed to involve something forceful that alters and transforms a person's consciousness, such that when Greg is not paranoid he feels he is 'living', the latter suggesting a sense of hope and unfolding future. Some aspects of extreme paranoia seem relevant to the concept of salience (Kapur, 2003), in that events seem full of meaning and importance; the state may also be understood as one of hyper-arousal (Porges, 2011).

Whether with extreme paranoia, or a less intense level, the participants still experienced a threatening untrustworthy world. From a phenomenological point of view, this might be understood as a transformation of what Ratcliffe (2008) calls 'existential feelings', that is, what it actually feels like to exist as oneself in a world in a specific way. An existential feeling is something in addition to any specific explicit thoughts, feelings, or narrations the person has, although these might influence each other. Psychosis can be seen as involving existential feelings and the sort here suggests a 'feeling of persecution', a feeling that one is not safe, that someone is deliberately plotting to carry out harm against oneself. Perhaps there is even a feeling of immanent terrible and perhaps cruel obliteration. While a person who does not have psychosis might entertain such ideas as a mere intellectual possibility, in paranoia the self and body are convulsed with a compelling sense of dreadful certainty.

As an individual experiences greater paranoia there are new certainties, increased suspicion, loss of trust, and whatever grip, fragile or otherwise, that the person had on his or her world before is pushed aside. In this state former 'common sense' of the everyday world, both assumptions and preverbal dispositions, is disconnected.

Further reflection will be given on the above interviews and themes in subsequent chapters. Chapter five will look at the topic of perceived aggression and violence and their relation to psychotic meanings. In chapter six a key focus will be on how participants experienced extreme states and sometimes changes in apparent identities of self and others. In chapter seven, I will focus on trust and the assumed everyday world.

Note

1 I am grateful to Wiley for granting me permission to reuse material from this article.

References

Bernstein, D.P., & Fink, L. (1998). *Childhood trauma questionnaire: A retrospective self-report manual.* San Antonio, TX: Psychological Corporation.

Cunningham, T., Hoy, K., & Shannon, C. (2016). Does childhood bullying lead to the development of psychotic symptoms? A meta-analysis and review of prospective studies. *Psychosis, 8,* 48–59.

Fisher, L.H., McGuffin, P., Boydell, J., Fearon, P., Craig, T.K., Dazzan, P., ... Morgan, C. (2014). Interplay between childhood physical abuse and familial risk in the onset of psychotic disorders. *Schizophrenia Bulletin, 40(6),* 1443–1451.

Kapur. S. (2003). Psychosis as a state of aberrant salience: A framework linking biology, phenomenology, and pharmacology in schizophrenia. *American Journal of Psychiatry, 160,* 13–23.

Porges, S.W. (2011). *The polyvagal theory: Neurophysiological foundations of emotions, attachment, communication, and self-regulation.* New York: Norton.

Ratcliffe, M. (2008). *Feelings of being: Phenomenology, psychiatry and the sense of reality.* Oxford: OUP.

Rhodes, J.E., & Healey, A.L. (2016). 'Many die in the hurricane': An interpretative phenomenological analysis of adults with psychosis and a history of physical abuse. *Clinical Psychology and Psychotherapy, 24(3),* 737–746.

Springer, K.W., Sheridan, J., Kuo, D., & Carnes, M. (2007). Long-term physical and mental health consequences of childhood physical abuse: Results from a large population-based sample of men and women. *Child Abuse and Neglect, 31*(5), 517–530.

Sugaya, L., Hasin, D.H., Olfson, M., Keng-Han, L., Grant, B.F., & Blanco, C. (2012). Child physical abuse and adult mental health: A national study. *Journal of Trauma Stress, 25*(4), 384–392.

3

SEXUAL ABUSE AND PSYCHOSIS

Introduction

Sexual abuse strikes at the core of human relations, destroying trust, care, respect, and leaving a multiple of negative consequences. This chapter focuses on the experiences of women who were diagnosed with psychosis and were subject to severe sexual abuse in childhood. The aim is to explore with the participants how they saw their lives and difficulties. The chapter draws on research presented in Rhodes, O'Neill, and Nel (2018).[1] First some relevant research findings are reviewed.

The long-term consequences of child sexual abuse

Considerable research has shown that child sexual abuse (CSA) has a wide range of damaging consequences in the lives of adult survivors. A review by Cashmore and Shackel (2013) highlighted the increased incidence of several psychiatric diagnoses among this population, including alcohol dependence,

DOI: 10.4324/9781003044956-3

social anxiety, PTSD, and psychosis. They also noted evidence of increased suicide attempts, sexual behaviours involving risk, difficulties in relationships, and potential re-victimisation. They concluded that the weight of evidence points to a causal relationship, though complex and involving many variables. Those with histories of CSA may suffer a range of long-term neurological changes (Teicher & Samson, 2016). Heim et al. (2013) looked at the specific influence of CSA on brain development and noted changes in areas of the cortex that are involved in sexual bodily experience.

Child sexual abuse and psychosis in adults

Quantitative research has begun to outline what may be specific causal connections; Bebbington et al. (2011) on the basis of their research suggested that there was in fact a specific causal link between CSA and psychosis. Bourgeois et al. (2018) looked at sexual abuse histories in teenagers and noted those abused were ten times more likely to receive a diagnosis of psychosis than teenagers without a history of abuse; furthermore, they noted that there was no gender difference in the prevalence of psychotic disorders. Marwaha and Bebbington (2015) explored the potential contributions of depression and anxiety to psychosis in those with sexual abuse, suggesting that these were important factors. All of these major studies point to the importance of sexual abuse as a causal factor in the manifestation of psychosis.

The participants

Recruitment did not specify gender at first, but after several months of being only referred women, we decided to focus on this group specifically. All of the women were known to local psychological and psychiatric services. Participants were included if they had a diagnosis of psychosis, had reported sexual abuse, and scored highly on sexual abuse but not physical abuse on the CTQ.

Participation in the research was voluntary and the interview was explained before the participants met the researcher. It was pointed out that the interview would not focus on details of the trauma itself, but rather the effects of trauma on their lives. Some basic characteristics of the participants are given in Table 3.1.

Table 3.1 Participant characteristics

Participant	Age at interview (years)	Ethnicity	Age at onset of abuse (years)	Approximate duration of abuse (years)	Diagnoses	Age of psychosis onset
Clare	35	White/English	8	7–8	Borderline personality disorder/ schizophrenia	Mid-20s
Jackie	35	Mixed race/ English	13	3–4	Bipolar affective disorder	Mid-20s
Irene	32	White/European	9	3–4	Anorexia–Schizoaffective disorder schizophrenia	19
Zoe	48	White/English	7	Unknown	Schizophrenia	Mid-30s
Toni	37	Black British	Below 8	4–8	Depression with psychotic features	Mid-20s
Sue	38	Black British	14 and late teens	2	Schizophrenia	Early 20s
Hasina	26	Asian/British	12	2	Schizophrenia	Early

The themes expressed by participants

Six main themes emerged from the analysis of the data: degradation of self; body-self entrapment; a sense of being different; unending struggle and depression; psychotic condemnations and abuse; and perception of links to the past.

Degradation of self

It was striking that four of the participants specifically described a feeling of being 'dirty'.

> I get nervous around people. I'm shy, I still feel dirty, no matter how many times I have a bath and that. I still feel that dirty feeling. (Jackie)

> ... coz they're always looking at, not all of them, but some men look at me in a way that makes me feel dirty. (Hasina)

The feeling of being 'dirty' appears to be felt in and on the body, and provokes bathing and hand washing. What is it to feel 'dirty'? When we think that others might perceive us as being less clean than society expects, our reaction can be of shame or disgust, of wanting to cover up or hide. The experience of these participants, however, is extreme and unending, something they somehow cannot change or ever 'wash off'. Hasina directly linked the experience to the sexual gaze of others, in particular older men. This experience seemed specific to a social situation involving men, whereas for Jackie it seemed to be about people in general. Irene expressed similar ideas concerning dirt:

> At the time I felt like I was a piece of crap basically. I must have been an evil bitch for this nasty thing to have happened to me.

She added a further extreme comment:

> I've said to other people, if I knew what my life was gonna be like, I would have strangled myself with the umbilical cord. And I'm not joking ...

The comments interconnect dirt, self-blame, and then the attitude that one's life should not have been lived. Perhaps to emphasise the suffering she feels, Irene presents an extreme and impossible scenario of the destruction of self involving going back in time. Whether this act is one of hate, or perhaps aims to prevent suffering, is left unsaid.

Toni stated that she did not hate herself, yet said:

> I don't see why I should be treated like something that comes off of somebody's shoe. I don't see why I should be treated that way. I don't deserve it.

Here she is probably referring to excrement, though it could be anything dirty. This is a metaphor of not only dirt, but something from the floor, and trodden underfoot. She is therefore seeing herself as beneath others, in a position of extreme inferiority and something rejected, for which others have disgust.

Three participants had less extreme expressions. Zoe said of herself:

> I'm feeling redundant and quite useless.

Zoe feared being made to feel 'humiliated', while two other participants stated that they had engaged in blaming themselves for their pasts:

> And so it's my fault, and so you blame yourself, and so for years and years and years of blaming yourself. (Clare)

> My self-esteem just went lower and lower over the years … I was feeling that maybe I was partly to blame even though I never instigated anything, umm, I felt, I felt guilty, everything sort of like rolled up into one. (Sue)

The 'blame' here might be understood as a less extreme experience of self-degradation. 'Blame' suggests an action carried out and is not so completely focused on the very core being of the person. Many feelings and thoughts, perhaps in contradiction, are 'rolled up', somehow all together in her.

In sum, all the participants experienced a sort of degradation, with degrees of self-judgement, which for most involved a feeling centred in the body. There is a cluster of overlapping experiences suggesting shame, guilt, and disgust.

Body–self entrapment

One participant, Clare, gave a vivid account of a bodily experience in childhood that was also experienced as an adult. She stated 'the way I was abused was quite crippling', then went on to say:

> I was saying it was crippling … that feeling I had as a child. Of being crippled. Sort of down trodden. I've had that in mental illness. But I've had it in sort of both extremes. I've had it like when I've felt totally uncrippled, you know? So that I actually own the whole world. And then I've had it so that literally my body is crippled. Where I can't walk properly. Or I can't see, or umm, hear things properly. Umm, it's sort of similar to being in that situation as a child. It feels, my body feels like it's … sort of shut down. Like there's nothing there, like it's all gone … It's like, when I'm ill, my, my legs totally change, my feet, my feet, do all sorts of things, umm, like clench up, and my big toe, toes all push out, and I can't walk properly.

She links feeling 'crippled' now as an adult directly to the feeling she had as a child. The feeling of being 'crippled', as an adult, occurs both in periods of psychosis and outside of these. When psychotic, and feeling the opposite of 'crippled', she owns the 'whole world', suggesting power and freedom. At other times her body loses its ability to move freely. It is as if she manifests in her body that she is not free, that she cannot even walk. For Clare there is often a feeling of being 'crippled', but during psychosis she begins to experience the feeling as a real and concrete state.

Jackie spoke of a time when she was 'spiralling out of control' and added:

> I mean I have a sense in my head of this sense of being trapped …

She went on to say that now that she is looking after her father, that is, the abuser:

> I feel trapped again … I feel all a bit trapped again. But I feel I'm in control this time more.

Here the idea of 'control' is explicitly mentioned. Perhaps for this participant being 'trapped' links to not having control over what happened to her. She emphasised her 'head' which might be the part of the body or self that should be in control. Zoe also had a sense of somehow being constricted:

> It's sort of erm, a mixture really, of thoughts and probably sen, strange bodily sensations. Sort of like, it's as if I'm cut off, around, like relating to my body ... Strange, it all seems to be related around my stomach ... like I'm constricted. It's tight and it's sort of umm, eh, very uncomfortable, very uncomfortable.

She added later:

> ... it's all in my body. It's peculiar, it's sort of like a numb feeling.

The experience combines disparate elements, 'thoughts', 'sensation', 'cut off', 'numb'. It is not clear how these cohere and in fact, perhaps they don't. Rather, it is a disturbing experience of fragmentation, and central to it is being 'constricted'. It seems a form of suffering experienced directly in the body itself but also involves thoughts and feelings.

Toni described the following:

> When I was a child, I didn't feel dead inside, but when I went into teenage years I began gradually to feel dead inside ... I feel as if I have no emotions. I can't express my anger. I have to keep my anger under control.

In spite of feeling 'dead' she suggested there was also:

> ... hatred and bitterness, that's intertwined.

Here being 'dead' seems related to the suppression of terrible feelings such as hate and 'bitterness'. We might think of these feelings as 'constricted', held back in the person. She feels dead yet has these extreme feelings which cannot be expressed.

The four accounts all suggest that somehow, in the body of the person, there is an experience of not being free, of not being able to express what might be powerful emotions and feelings. Two clearly relate the feeling as beginning in childhood, while a third suggested her teenage years. One participant was able to describe how a feeling from childhood is transformed in adult psychosis.

A sense of being different

In discussing their adult lives, most of the participants articulated a sense that they were different from others and found themselves isolated and cut off. Linked to this was a perception that others were not to be trusted, and some mentioned the difficulty of intimate sexual relations. Zoe said:

> I feel like I stand out, sort of stand out like a sore thumb sometimes, you know, sort of like I'm the odd one out.

The following were similar comments made by others:

> No, most of the time I feel the odd one out. (Jackie)

> Like I see it, like I'm on the outside looking in, and I don't like what I see. (Irene)

> Experience has taught me that fitting in doesn't work. (Toni)

Six of the participants made such comments: a common image is that one is apart from the others. Clare did not make an explicit comment but did emphasise that during a long period she had 'isolated' herself and that, concerning her family:

> They find it difficult to understand where I'm coming from. And so I find it difficult to trust them.

A picture emerged of participants seeing themselves as isolated and different. They do not fit into what they construe as the everyday world. Whether the imagined world of others is good or otherwise is sometimes left open, but at other times the other is depicted as untrustworthy. That participants could not trust others was mentioned explicitly by five. Toni stated:

Well, I've come to the stage I can't trust anybody because you put your trust in someone only for them to betray your trust. They, they, I mean, nobody, nobody knows what goes on in the mind. Coz it might be legit, but they might have ulterior motives.

Others present a surface which conceals ulterior motives. Six of the participants explicitly mentioned intimate relationships and all reported great difficulties. Sue stated:

I just find it difficult to establish relationships because there will always be ulterior motives.

Hasina had had one long relationship, but mentioned this difficulty:

... even when I was with the person that I loved, the boyfriend, I'll watch the way that he'll do things, the way he's got my clothes. If before we got intimate, my clothes will be on the bed. And he'll just chuck it, he'll fling it off. I used to get angry ... it used to make me think, you're flinging off me.

During intimacy she felt he was mistreating her, and in her distress, she sees herself and her clothes as equivalent, in fact her clothes are her. As if the situation so disturbed her that the boundaries of what exists have broken down, and he therefore has really shown hostility or indifference to her and not just her clothes. What might have been just a figure of speech, here a metonymy, has been taken as literally true. Clearly being close was fraught with such extreme difficulties that the boundaries of the self were metamorphosed. Zoe stated:

And the dreadful loneliness and isolation and at the same time finding it difficult to get close to people.

Being the 'odd one out' was experienced alongside great loneliness. In sum, the participants felt they themselves were different, and this was in a world where others could not be trusted and often had other, usually negative, motives.

Unending struggle and depression

All the participants mentioned a great number of problems concerning relationships, work, and daily life. Clare stated:

> Basically, I haven't been able to live a normal life. I've been very depressed, sad and depressed, and couldn't see any way through it. I could never see a way through it.

And Jackie:

> Just you can't seem to feel happy in yourself at all. You're just down all the time and everything is a struggle. That's about it really.

In a similar vein, Sue mentioned depression and then said:

> I'm more quiet, more withdrawn, and sometimes I feel like I've got the whole world on my shoulder ... like even though I know other people have problems but I feel like my one's a big problem.

Not only are the participants feeling depressed, and also list several negative emotions such as feeling down, sad, worried, at the same time there is a sense of being overwhelmed by things and having no hope for change. The experience seems constant for some, as Jackie says above, while for others such as Zoe there is some variability:

> I get times when I'm really really down. I get, I feel confusion, forgetfulness, forget things. Umm, I'm constantly worried about my looks deteriorating.

And in one sweeping comment, Toni stated when asked about her life:

> Broken, spiritually, mentally, emotionally.

The participants had a multitude of both practical and emotional problems in their daily lives. In addition, there is a sense of unending difficulties, that life is a complete struggle. Whether the struggles 'cause' or contribute to the misery, or in fact, that repeated depression has led to difficulties (or both simultaneously) was not clarified.

Psychotic condemnations and abuse

All the participants spoke openly of 'voices' or times in their lives when they regarded themselves as being 'paranoid'. These were the actual words of the participants: whether a voice or delusional situation was real or a product of the person's mind (i.e., according to the participants themselves) was very variable and often unclear. The aim here however is not to settle such issues but to focus on the content as given.

The most common overarching theme was of some sort of condemnation combined with threats: the condemnation in all cases seemed to originate from people or entities external to the person. The condemnation concerned something being wrong with the person, for example, that the person was evil. Some condemnation focused on issues of sexual abuse activity, while other condemnations were vague. In the following there is first a focus on more general condemnation linked with harm, then later condemnation linked with specific ideas of sexual abuse.

Five of the participants mentioned ideas relating to condemnation and harm. Clare heard voices:

> And then the voices were 'She doesn't even feel guilty about what she's done'. You know 'Look at her, she totally doesn't care about what she's done' and eh, I'm 'Well I would care if I knew what it was'. You know? And so the conversation goes on. And the whole time the conversation is going on, you're having all these thoughts. And, and to the point where, umm. Where, where you're actually now thinking 'well, if I'm that evil, I must, I must just kill myself now' you know because I can't be evil.

There seems to be a tortured conversation going on internally within the person. She seems first to overhear a conversation between voices that point out her lack of guilt at what she has done. There follows a sort of question and answer within the person: she wonders what she could have done, but then reaches a sort of conclusion, that she must be evil and so must take action. Toni stated without elaboration:

> I have intrusive suicidal thoughts.

And about others:

> I still think everyone is out to get me … humiliate, degrade me.

While three participants had ideas of suicide, for three others the issue was of more general harm. Hasina stated:

... they just laugh at me, and they say to me they want me to hurt myself ... and if I don't do it they'll keep going on at me, going on at me, and when I start screaming or banging my head on the wall they're laughing louder and louder.

What might happen to Sue was left vague but suggested something negative done against her:

... the voices are telling me there's repercussions to follow afterwards.

In the following themes self harm and explicit sexual abuse related topics are combined. Jackie came to believe that she was taken to be a paedophile:

I felt like it was the press and the television were all on me and they all thought I was this paedophile.

And, as she listened to the voices, she had almost killed herself:

I thought that I was a paedophile, and that everybody knew what I was. And they thought. No I didn't think I was a paedophile, I thought everybody thought I was ... And I thought I was gonna go to prison, and that I should hang myself or put myself under a train or ... and the voices were telling me I should do that. But it was me, and my self-belief 'but I'm not', that stopped me from doing that.

Reading the passage suggests that the main issue for Jackie was, did others believe she is a paedophile? Yet the fact she first says she thought she was one could be taken to show the sort of confusion she might have experienced at the time. The theme of sexual abuse is clearly present in the issue of being a 'paedophile' but here the person, the one who had been a victim of abuse, is led to believe that she is the abuser. In this episode, it seems that for a while she experienced herself as having a changed identity at least in the way she was perceived by others. Facing up to this situation, she considered killing herself, something the voices reinforced, but her 'self belief' stopped it. These comments suggest turmoil, a great struggle within the person. Another participant, Zoe, recounted a recurring incident:

... there is a neighbour next door, and I thought he called me a paedophile.

Again, the abused person is now called the abuser. Sue was subject to endless and terrible insults by voices:

> ... you're a fool, oh, and you're a dirty bitch.

When asked if she meant the abuse, she confirmed this. She also stated:

> ... it's like, I imagine whatever I've done, other people will follow, will know what I've done. So that's how the voices come about, come from.

Irene was an exception in that her psychotic content did not seem focused on condemnation; however, there were issues of abuse. She recounted an extraordinary incident in which she heard the voice of the abuser, but also felt his presence:

> ... my grandfather came to me and said he did what he did, he sexually abused me because he was sexually abused himself ...

This was followed by:

> It came into, he came into me.

When asked how she had felt she stated:

> It was frightening, but it also felt, ... umm, it felt, healing, not in the sense that I had him there, but for him to explain why he was a bastard basically.

And later others saw his 'presence':

> And they said 'look, there's the grandfather, you can see the grandfather in her'. And he was. I don't know how many years he was dead ... They could see his presence in me.

For Irene, these experiences had great significance: she was clear she thought it had really occurred but realised that others would see it as imagined.

In psychotic episodes the relation to abuse is usually not a simple one of recollecting episodes: for Irene her psychotic experiences in a sense were an addition to what happened in the past, a sort of continuation and al-teration of the narrative. The range of possible thematic alterations seems open. Whatever the permutation, the topic of abuse returns transformed.

In sum, experiences which the participants themselves described as voices, or sometimes paranoid thinking, concentrated on themes of con-demnation, sometimes relating to sexual abuse (four participants), sometimes condemnation with more general threats (six participants). The way they related to the topic of abuse was however complex and open.

Condemnation involved insulting contempt, or degrees of self harm. For several participants the topic of abuse, or the attacking conversation of voices, activated the person to have sequences of disturbed thinking or a sort of tormented dialogue within the self.

Perception of links to the past

All the participants considered that, in a variety of ways, the past had had a major influence on their adult suffering. In contrast, however, most did not suggest that the abuse led to psychosis or, to be more precise, that the abuse had created the voices or paranoia (or what we from the outside might see as delusions). Discussing how she had suffered types of eating disorder, Irene stated:

> When I went into psychiatric care is because of my past. It's got everything to do with my past. I was anorexic, because I had no control of my life. Umm, I wasn't believed with what was happening when I was younger.

Hasina was able to link to several problems:

> I think it's mainly my stammer, and my cleansing-ness and my thoughts.

However, when specifically asked about the 'spirits', she said she did not know if this linked to the abuse, but then went on to mention that she thought her mother had been put under a curse.

Jackie also saw connections with adult suffering and abuse. She de-scribed how she drank excessive amounts of alcohol:

> I think just to blank things out. Make things feel happy, in myself and blank out the night times. I used to drink until I could fall asleep with no problems ...

Jackie was the only participant to consider explicitly whether abuse had created her psychosis, but even she prevaricated:

> I've got a feeling they've got a link. It's either that or it's genetic. But I should think, I think there's a link. And my partner thinks there's a link between that as well.

It would therefore seem that the idea came from someone else. She knew a sibling and a relative who had psychosis, and this might have led her to consider genetic factors.

In sum, all could see links between abuse and suffering, but the psychosis itself was not included in that explanatory frame. Sometimes the 'spirits' or voices reacted to the abuse, or knew about it, but they had not been created by it.

Overview

The study of adult women survivors of CSA who experienced psychosis suggested that they suffered from long-term feelings of 'degradation', sometimes accompanied by feelings of self-blame, sometimes of being 'dirty'; of feeling that their bodies were trapped or 'crippled', as if disconnected but also feeling held back or restricted. They saw themselves as 'different' from others and felt isolated: intimate relationships were rare or difficult.

They experienced several psychiatric symptoms and a wide range of social and practical difficulties, cumulating in a sense that life is full of depression and struggle. The experiences participants described as 'voices' or 'paranoia' were marked by a general theme of condemnation expressed in two subordinate themes. The first subordinate theme involved a reference to sexually abusive activities, though not as a reliving of past experiences. The second subordinate theme was of harm with condemnation, sometimes with an imperative to commit self-harm, including suicide.

Three participants in a phase of severe psychosis underwent a disturbance in their sense of identity, of who or what they were, in that they believed that others perceived them as 'paedophiles', and Clare was tormented about whether she was 'evil'. For all the participants, the sense of condemnation seemed deeper than just an idea, or a specific emotion, but rather an existential feeling (Ratcliffe, 2008) of being in a condemning world, an outsider and in danger.

Clearly the seven women suffered enormously throughout their lives, and themes of sexual abuse were manifest both in psychotic content and in other experiences. It is striking that two of the themes, that is, self-degradation and body self-entrapment, strongly focused on a distorted experience of the body. The extremity of Jackie's lost of control over the movements of her body could well be seen a type of dissociation (Van der Hart, Niejenhuis, & Steele, 2006), though such a diagnosis had not been made.

In terms of how the women suffered outside the specific area of psychosis, it seems fairly clear that these women were comparable to other women who had been sexually abused but who did not have psychosis, that is, they had problems with relationships but also with mood, depression, anxiety, and maintaining an occupation. The women stated very clearly that the abuse they had suffered had led to a range of extreme difficulties in their adult life such as depression or eating disorders, but in general they did not see their psychotic experiences, in particular voices and paranoia, as being created by their abuse. This of course this has therapeutic implications in that not only do individuals not see parallels between these areas concerning psychosis but, in fact, such links might well be resisted or rejected by participants. This topic will be returned to in later chapters on therapy.

Note

1 I am grateful to Wiley for granting me permission to reuse material from this article.

References

Bebbington, P.E., Jonas, S., Kuipers, E., King, M., Cooper, C., Brugha, ... Jenkins, R. (2011). Sexual abuse and psychosis: data from an English National Survey. *British Journal of Psychiatry, 199*(1), 29–37.

Bourgeois, C., Lecomte, T., & Daigneault, I. (2018). Psychotic disorders in sexually abused youth: a prospective matched-cohort study. *Schizophrenia Research, 199*, 123–127.

Cashmore, J., & Shackel, R. (2013). *The long-term effects of child sexual abuse* (CFCA Paper No. 11). Melbourne: IFS.

Heim, C.M., Mayberg, H.S., Mletzko, T., Nemeroff, C.B., & Pruessner, J.C. (2013). Decreased cortical representation of genital somatosensory field after childhood sexual abuse. *American Journal of Psychiatry, 170,* 616–623.

Marwaha, S., & Bebbington, P. (2015). Mood as a mediator of the link between child sexual abuse and psychosis. *Social Psychiatry and Psychiatric Epidemiology, 50,* 661–663.

Ratcliffe, M. (2008). *Feelings of being: Phenomenology, psychiatry and the sense of reality.* Oxford: OUP.

Rhodes, J.E., O'Neill, N., & Nel, P. (2018). Psychosis and sexual abuse: An interpretative phenomenological analysis. *Clinical Psychology and Psychotherapy, 25,* 540–549.

Teicher, M.H., & Samson, J.A. (2016). Annual research review: Enduring neurobiological effects of childhood abuse and neglect. *Journal of Child Psychology and Psychiatry, 57*(3), 241–266.

Van der Hart, O., Niejenhuis, E., & Steele, K. (2006). *The haunted self: Structural dissociation and the treatment of chronic traumatisation.* New York: Norton.

4

REFUGEES AND PSYCHOSIS

Introduction

This chapter describes the experiences of adult refugees and asylum seekers diagnosed with psychosis and who had experienced trauma in their country of origin. In contrast to the previous two chapters, the focus here is on the effects of trauma undergone by adults. The participants for the research presented in Rhodes, Parrett, and Mason (2016)[1] were recruited with histories of at least one traumatic life event involving political violence such as the experience of torture, war, or political killings. The findings will be presented following an overview of the evidence base concerning psychosis in survivors of political violence.

Mental health problems of refugees

Refugees have a higher incidence of mental health problems than the general population (Fazel, Wheeler & Danesh, 2005). Rates of post-traumatic

DOI: 10.4324/9781003044956-4

stress disorder (PTSD) in particular are shown to be elevated (Lavik et al., 1996; Turner et al., 2003), and anxiety and depressive disorders are also common. Studies measuring rates of psychotic disorders are rare, even though there have been indications for some time of an increased incidence (Eitinger, 1959).

Psychosis in survivors of political violence

Parrett and Mason (2010) found fourteen studies to review with information relating to psychosis in refugee populations. From this limited evidence, they concluded that refugees are at an increased risk of psychosis, and that psychological trauma may have played a key role in many cases. One study of refugees and residents of the former Yugoslavia (Jankovic et al., 2013) found that war trauma was associated with a sixfold increase in the probability of a diagnosis of a psychotic disorder. Kroll et al. (2011) recorded an unusually high rate of 80% psychosis prevalence in 130 male Somali refugees aged 18–30 years. The authors tentatively pointed to the almost universal major exposure to trauma, dislocation, and starvation in the war of 1991, together with subsequent drug use and cultural role expectations, as all potentially contributing to psychosis onset.

Trauma, psychosis, and hallucinations

Hallucinations were a common symptom in the participants described in this chapter and may be defined as sensory perceptions that do not result from an external stimulus but have a compelling reality. They are conceptualised distinctly from intrusive memories or flashbacks as seen in PTSD, although parallels have been proposed in the potentially trauma-based genesis of these symptoms. Romme and Escher (1989) found 70% of voice hearers developed their hallucinations following a traumatic event. Hardy et al. (2005) found that in a group of individuals who had experienced trauma with a diagnosis of schizophrenia or related disorders, 12.5% had hallucinations with similar content to their trauma and 45% hallucinations with similar themes. These findings suggest that plausible causal links can be made between trauma and hallucinations, perhaps in a way that parallels the more obvious ones between traumatic experiences and PTSD.

The participants

Four adult refugees and three asylum seekers living in the UK, and diagnosed with psychosis in a psychiatric setting, participated in this study. Six participants were from sub-Saharan Africa and one from North Africa. An interpreter was used with one participant (Frederic). Demographic and clinical characteristics of the participants are summarised in Table 4.1. All participants reported experiencing auditory hallucinations, along with other mental health symptoms (commonly of psychotic, affective, and post-traumatic disorders).

The interview schedule was based on the authors' clinical experience in the area and the relevant literature (e.g., Halabi, 2005). The areas explored were: how life was for the person at the present time; any difficulties in general; the experience of voices and other features described in the medical notes; and ideas concerning the future. Given the possibility of raising unmanageable feelings during the interview, participants were informed both during recruitment and prior to the first interview that they would not be asked specifically about any previous traumatic experiences. Ethical approval was granted by the local research ethics committee.

Themes expressed in the experiences of adult survivors of political violence who have been diagnosed with psychosis

Seven themes emerged from the analysis of the participants' accounts: bleak agitated immobility; trauma-related voices and visions; fear and

Table 4.1 Participant details

Name	Gender	Age (years)	Asylum Status	Diagnosis
Frederic	M	39	Refugee	Depression with psychotic features
Togar	M	29	Appeal	Paranoid schizophrenia
Lionel	M	37	Appeal	PTSD and psychosis
Sando	M	26	Appeal	PTSD and psychotic symptoms
Belvie	F	30	Refugee	PTSD and psychotic symptoms
Saacid	M	39	Refugee	PTSD and psychotic illness
Amine	M	43	Refugee	Paranoid schizophrenia

mistrust of others; the sense of a broken self; the pain of losing everything; despair and recurrent breakdown; and the attraction of death.

Bleak-agitated immobility

All interviewees described a sense of having no future, of losing hope, and of being in a difficult, distressing situation. They expressed feeling that they were not moving forward with their lives. Sando stated:

> It's like I'm on the track running. I am an athlete running, but I never see the finish line. Other people run on the track, they have a finish line, even if they are running a marathon. But I have been running since … I never see a finish line, so I don't know how long I will continue to run.

By likening his existence to a never-ending race, Sando stresses a struggle he cannot win and to which there is no end in sight. He is moving, running, yet getting nowhere as if stuck. It is a strange place, where others get somewhere but not him. For three of the participants, their wait in the asylum process was a concern, but all the participants expressed similar ideas of being immobile:

> I was 25 and had dreamed to find a good job and career. But everything stopped because of what I went through. I'm trying to do things, but I can't, it's hard for me.

Here Belvie is locating the source of her problems in what happened to her, with the trauma she had experienced having stopped her life. The stopping of 'everything' suggests all she values, not just specific activities. She tries, but it leads to no result. For Amine, this feeling goes even further:

> I think life for me has become like a stranger. I cannot deal with her. I can't work, I can't have a good job. Day after day is just the same, like a routine.

He added:

> I feel like I'm finished. There's no life, there's no future, there's no anything anymore. I think everything is going to become like darkness.

Life for him is now a 'stranger', someone unknown, which for him links to not being able to deal with things, not being able to work, and having an unchanging routine. Unlike Sando, he is not even running. He is finished, and the darkness suggests a pervasive nihilism has overtaken him. Though he is biologically alive, his sense of having a life is gone and all he now expects is darkness.

The experience of being a traumatised refugee appears to place the person in a bleak landscape of pain and fruitless struggle. With no hope, and in spite of great effort, there is a feeling that one is going nowhere. It is as if a refugee struggles to find a home, a safe place in which to belong, but cannot arrive there.

Trauma-related voices and visions

All the participants experienced voices, and five reported various visual phenomena. It was striking that six related what they heard to episodes of trauma. Frederic described hearing voices similar to those heard at the time of his arrest:

> I hear these voices saying 'Stop, arrest him. Kill him. Kill him'. Like the soldiers used to say in my country.

Three participants heard voices related to specific episodes involving being attacked, while three heard voices that involved transformations of trauma-related experience. Sando heard his dead mother calling:

> She is telling me 'come join us'. So for me, she came to get me... they are trying to communicate with me, maybe they are trying to send me a message.

Sando believed that his mother was speaking to him from beyond the grave following her murder. He assumed his mother, even in death, was making a suggestion to help him. This indicates that he still feels a deep connection to her. Belvie reported a mixture of voices, both trauma related and recent:

> Some voice I have it's like from the past. But some of them are not from the past. I don't know. Sometimes it's like a voice of the thing that was done to me when I was back home, when I was tortured. Sometimes I hear the voice of that person.

Whereas Sando hears the voice of someone loved, Belvie hears a persecutor. However, it is not just the voice of the person, but of the 'thing' done to her. Both 'torture' and 'torturer' have a 'voice'. The torture has been personified. Her fractured references perhaps reflect a fragmentation in the terrible experience and its recollection.

Five participants reported a diverse range of disturbing visual phenomena. All five had sometimes thought that what was seen existed outside themselves, and of these, four had thematic links to trauma. Sando heard and also saw his dead mother:

My mum was in one of those interviews and it was her on the TV.

He also saw her on the street:

I run after the woman, calling her '…', … you know, the woman turned back, and look at me and it wasn't her.

Here Sando saw the person he longed to see, but in contrast, Lionel saw threatening things: at one time he often saw what he took to be soldiers from his country.

Saacid also had threatening visions and spoke of seeing the 'spirits' of those he had seen die in war situations:

Yeah [pause] yeah their spirit.,

going on to say that this was 'some country man' and that they looked very 'scary'.

Amine spoke of terrible nightmares of seeing his brother covered in blood and asking for help, but he also spoke of seeing a picture on a wall in the hospital:

It's like a man but it's not a man like but not an animal …

And further that it somehow came out of the picture: he then wavered over whether he regarded this as real or otherwise. This experience did not seem to link thematically to the past in any obvious direct way, except perhaps as a general experience of terror and the other.

The two main themes of voices and visions were attackers and lost loved ones. These were manifest in a very wide range of auditory and visual phenomena, often taken to be real and external to the person. The majority saw thematic links, either directly from experienced episodes, or involving meaningful transformations.

Fear and mistrust of others

Five participants expressed variations of interpersonal fear and mistrust. Amine felt terror when surprised, even by friendly others; he linked his fear of people to the period when he was persecuted and then said:

> If someone comes behind and touches me like that, I feel here like a stone in my chest, here… and now sometimes just a noise gives me a shock.

It seemed that fear transformed his body, such that he experienced something painful, hard, and destructive within him. Belvie also had a terror of others, for example, when someone looked at her on the bus she thought:

> Who is it, what he will do for, what he will do? Maybe he will kill me or something like that.

She appeared to have lost everyday trust, and instead expected violence. Sando stated a lack of trust explicitly:

> They might trust me. But I don't trust them.

They were aware that these reactions started in the contexts of trauma, yet knowing this did not stop the participants having immediate, bodily felt fearful perceptions of others. Everyday trust in others had collapsed.

The sense of a broken self

Several participants described how they felt that they had changed in a very general and extensive sense, as if their self had undergone a global and perhaps permanent alteration. Amine stated:

> ... and sometimes I feel like I am broken. Everything is broken and I can't find how to make it better ... just my face and my pictures are still this man, inside I am totally different.

His face, perhaps in the mirror, and the photos he saw of himself, suggested that he was the same person, yet inside he felt completely different. It was as if he was no longer the same being or person, even if others from the outside did not see the difference. The participants listed several aspects of themselves which they found to be different:

> My emotional state has changed and my personality has changed, ... I really haven't been alright (Frederic)

> I can think today. It's not it's my thinking, it's not the way, you know, I was. (Belvie)

Different participants emphasised different changes, and these included ways of thinking, of being emotional, but also a general sense of not being the same person. To understand, we need to imagine not just an isolated trauma, but how one then finds one's self different, broken, and unable to find a way to mend.

The pain of losing everything

Participants spoke about their lives before refugee status, in which they were just 'normal' and 'did everyday things', and compared this with their current situation. They often seemed to look back with yearning on a happy and stable past that contrasted radically with their current situation.

> We used to fit all together, we had no problems, it was really good ... I do suffer and I miss a lot of things. (Frederic)

> No matter where you be, no matter what you be, there is no place like home ... I feel like lonely, I feel like hopeless, that I'm useless. (Togar)

The degree of loss for these participants is difficult for us to grasp: they have lost their worlds. A new location or role does not replace 'home', that place of familiarity and warmth. The loss of others, and even what has happened, is still unknown, leading to unending sadness:

For my family, yeah, because I don't know where are they … when to see them. Whether they alive or dead. So the thing, you feel like you sad … all the time. (Lionel)

The past was good, not only in relation to family, friends, and work, but also a sense of belonging, of 'fit' and of 'home', while in the present all they felt was its absence. We are perhaps not really aware of how much we rely on our everyday connections until they are ripped asunder. For some, the pain was made worse by not knowing what had happened to loved ones.

Despair and recurrent breakdown

All of the participants described being in states of distress, suffering, and depression, which at times became more intense. This could occur while reflecting on the past, the present, or a challenging future. Frederic presented his suffering in a resigned and quiet way, yet full of profound feeling:

I have a lot of regrets so sometimes I just stay at home and I just cry and tears just come.

As if he has only to withdraw to the solitude of his home and then the tears 'just come', as if he carried these somewhere inside ready to fall. Togar said concerning his ongoing situation:

When I start to think about it I get depressed.

He said he felt like this in particular because he saw how others lived and that he could not live what he regarded as a normal life anymore, and that this actually felt like 'torture'. He added that he felt:

… hopeless, that I'm useless, I see like God doesn't like me.

Not only that there is no hope, but he is rejected by the being which he believes guides the world: he is therefore completely abandoned. He went on to say:

I'm feeling pain like … I feel like dying when I have the current like shock.

The comparison he makes here is extraordinary and difficult to interpret: he seems to be pointing to some kind of actual emotional pain felt in his body. It reminds us that emotional pain is not something just abstract and mental, but felt, something that torments the body, or rather, the body-self. Physical pain and emotional pain are not separate. There is also a possible echo of how he might have been treated and tortured, although he did not go on to comment on that. Lionel stated that his moments of suffering were:

it feels like you don't have life, you don't have hope

, and that this left him,

sad all the time.

He went on to add, when thinking about his lost family that he had:

too many thoughts in your heart

, and later,

you have things you think in your heart which is paining you

Here again thought, feeling, and physical embodiment are experienced as a unity, and the thoughts and the pain are located in his heart. It is easy to assume that this purely metaphorical, but that would be to miss how in his experience all these elements are fused, and how this mixture of features characterises the experience. Sando stated that at those moments when he began to think about things:

100% there is no hope for me I break down badly … every time I think about that, it has the same impact, the same breakdown, stressed, loss of appetite, start having nightmare. But most of the time if I'm not thinking about what's gonna happen in the future. If I don't talk about the past or get myself too much worry, I will be fine. But if I start having all this talk of asking myself the question about what's gonna happen tomorrow, or if they say and I can't stay here we can send you back home, you know, I start to feel vulnerable and very very depressed.

The participants described trying to cope, and yet sometimes finding themselves thinking too much and feeling overwhelmed: disturbing thoughts and feelings could concern the past, present, and future. At such times the participants experienced great pain, extreme emotions, an excess of thoughts, and a pervasive sense of hopelessness.

The attraction of death: to live or die

Participants spoke openly about the seemingly insurmountable struggle to survive, and the suicide attempts they had made; while at other times expressing their hopes and wishes to continue and build a new life in a new country. For some, in diverse ways, death appeared as attractive. Sando heard his family suggest that it would be better to be dead:

> These people telling me to join them, it's better place over there you know, to telling me 'Listen, why are you here for'?

However, Sando also expressed concern that he might not be able to put up with his life any more:

> The worst part is I keep harming myself...and you know knocking my head to the wall, kinda too much stuff in there, you know, I just want to open my head and finish with this.

In this tortured image, Sando describes how he is trying to get on, yet represents his head as a burden, full of harmful stuff. It is as if he is fragmented and the parts are in conflict. He thinks that he can only stop this by 'opening' his head; he would escape yet die. Togar also saw death as attractive at times:

> When I be, when I get this problem I say, 'Oh is better for me to be dying down there' is better for me.

In contrast for Belvie, the ideas of taking her life seemed to represent an end point of trying, that she just could not carry on:

I've tried to harm myself maybe four, five times because I didn't have like a ... the thing ... for life, there's nothing. And it was very hard ...

In spite of the above negative attitudes and feelings, all except Amine were able to express some positive goals. Frederic, for example, said:

I want to integrate into this country. I want to have qualifications and work here.

Others mentioned reasons for living such as their religion or wanting to continue their family lines. Given the extremity of what had been experienced, and now finding themselves in a strange world, often not welcoming, it is perhaps not surprising that individuals' wish to live had become conflicted with a desire to escape.

Overview

The participants described terrifying perceptions often related to a traumatic past, though not usually a direct reliving of it. They made efforts to change, yet felt stuck as if their lives were not moving forwards: this was coupled with a yearning for the past, when life was normal and good for them. All expressed distress, saying they were sometimes depressed, felt hopeless, that they cried, feeling sadness and anger. Two stated they actually felt physical pain at such times. While some managed to form social networks, the majority experienced fear and mistrust of others. Some experienced a sense that they were not the person they had been in the past. All experienced moments when death seemed attractive as an escape from further suffering. Participants expressed a wish to die, held in tension with their wish to live and build a purposeful and worthwhile life. These conflicting ideas were similar to those expressed by Sudanese youth refugees is the study of Goodman (2004).

Several participants vividly expressed a sense that they had somehow been 'broken' or 'damaged' by their experience: this is consistent with reports of a connection between trauma and changes in the experience of self (Herman, 1992). Feeling stuck and without hope for the future was a powerful and common theme: similar themes have been discussed in previous literature concerning refugees (Tribe, 2002) and people experiencing psychosis (Warman et al., 2004). It was striking that the profound sense of having no future, of not moving forwards in a normal way, was found for both those who had been granted refugee status and for those who were awaiting an asylum decision. In everyday life many of us take for granted a sense of life unfolding and of being able to make future plans. For our participants, this sense of life had been torn from them, and had not been replaced by the feeling of living in a safe place.

Given the participants' histories of persecution and exposure to violence, it is not surprising that mistrust was found to be a distinctive theme. For some it was expressed by a very tentative approach to new friends, rarely trusting others, and only slowly building a relationship. This is consistent with much of the evidence relating to the loss of trust following trauma (Herman, 1992). For others it was yet more profound and led to isolation and a general mistrust of those they met both socially and those in the healthcare system. Gross (2004) noted similar problems of trust of services by refugees in Switzerland.

Napo et al. (2012) found that patients with a diagnosis of schizophrenia from West Africa often used the concept of 'spirits' as an explanatory model. While some of our participants described phenomena that seemed spirit-like (Sando, Saacid), the more common description suggested attackers, or even soldiers, though their status as living or dead was not clarified. The severe trauma of war and political violence may explain some pervasive themes for the present sample.

Ratcliffe et al. (2014) argued that any personal project for the future involves trusting others: work and family life requires cooperative actions and therefore trust. They suggest that this may account for 'a sense of foreshortened future' in those with trauma, since the possibility of trust has been destroyed. Our participants clearly expressed this sense of getting nowhere and having nothing ahead of them. They had lost trust in others and in addition found themselves in a new and difficult cultural landscape. They experienced a sort of double alienation. The very feeling of existence (Ratcliffe, 2008) of the world and self had dramatically altered: they displayed a painful awareness of something lost, perhaps a previously taken-for-granted sense of existing with others in a safe and predictable world. In contrast in the present they found themselves in a bleak static world shorn of benign possibility, cut off from others, at the edge of danger, and strangely not the selves that they had been.

Within psychiatric classifications, hallucinations are formally separated from post-traumatic memory intrusions such as 'flashbacks': the interviewees in our study, however, reported a spectrum of experiences that included the voices of past perpetrators, the voices of others more recently encountered, but also nightmares and flashbacks. Some authors (Morrison, Frame, & Larkin, 2003) refer to this overlap as 'traumatic psychosis', and this seems an apposite description of the experiences reported here. The trauma-related intrusions did not appear to be relived experiences in the classic 'PTSD' sense, but rather to be engrossing and believable perceptions 'flavoured' by past trauma. It was clear that at times, these perceptions were experienced as being externally generated: this is usually taken to be diagnostically indicative of psychosis rather than PTSD. However, Herman (1992) suggested that those who have undergone extreme trauma may have symptoms and patterns that do not fit well into conventional classifications. The themes of enduring fear and distrust, as well as the stuckness and hopelessness seen in the participants, resembled closely the symptoms described by Herman (1992) as 'complex PTSD'. Some also mentioned self-injury and wishing for death: behaviours and emotions also reported following sustained and severe traumatic events. The findings indicate that it may be a diagnostic mistake to interpret hallucinations in the context of extreme war trauma as pathognomonic of 'schizophrenia': that rather these may exist at a boundary between post-traumatic dissociation and psychosis. Conventional Western diagnostic categories do not seem well constructed to account for our participants' experiences. Given the findings here, perhaps a fitting description of our participants' difficulties would be 'complex PTSD with perceptual disturbances'.

In the following chapters further features of refugees with trauma and psychosis will be analysed but also comparisons made with those who suffered childhood abuse. The potentially overlapping but different pathways from abuse to psychosis will be discussed in chapter seven.

Note

1 I am grateful to Taylor & Francis for granting me permission to reuse material from this article.

References

Eitinger, L. (1959). The incidence of mental disease among refugees in Norway. *Journal of Mental Science, 105*, 326–328.

Fazel, M., Wheeler, J., & Danesh, J. (2005). Prevalence of serious mental disorder in 7000 refugees resettled in western countries: A systematic review. *The Lancet, 365*(9467), 1309–1314.

Goodman, J.H. (2004). Coping with trauma and hardship among unaccompanied refugee youths from Sudan. *Qualitative Health Research, 14*(9), 1177–1196.

Gross, C.S. (2004). Struggling with imaginaries of trauma and trust: The refugee experience in Switzerland. *Cultural Medicine and Psychiatry, 28*, 151–167.

Halabi, J.O. (2005). Nursing research with refugee clients: A call for more qualitative approaches. *International Nursing Review, 52*(4), 270–275.

Hardy, A., Fowler, D., Freeman, D., Smith, B., Steel, C., Evans, J., ... Dunn, G. (2005). Trauma and hallucinatory experience in psychosis. *Journal of Nervous & Mental Disease: 193*(8), 501–507

Herman, J.L. (1992). *Trauma and recovery*. New York: Basic Books.

Jankovic, J., Bremner, S., Bogic, M., Lecic-Tosevski, D., Ajdukovic, D., Franciskovic, T., ... Priebe, S. (2013). Trauma and suicidality in war affected communities. *European Psychiatry, 28*, 514–520.

Kroll, J., Yusuf, A.I., & Fujiwara, K. (2011). Psychoses, PTSD, and depression in Somali refugees in Minnesota. *Social Psychiatry and Psychiatric Epidemiology, 46*, 481–493.

Lavik, N.J., Hauff, E., Skrondal, A., & Solberg, Ø. (1996). Mental disorder among refugees and the impact of persecution and exile: some findings from an out-patient population. *British Journal of Psychiatry, 169*, 726–732.

Morrison, A.P., Frame, L., & Larkin, W. (2003). Relationships between trauma and psychosis: A review and integration. *British Journal of Clinical Psychology, 42*, 331–353.

Parrett, N.S., & Mason, O.J. (2010). Refugees and psychosis: A review of the literature. *Psychosis, 2*, 111–121.

Napo, F., Heinz, A., & Auckenthaler, A. (2012). Explanatory models and concepts of West African Malian patients with psychotic symptoms. *European Psychiatry, 27*(2), 44–49.

Ratcliffe, M. (2008). *Feelings of Being: Phenomenology, Psychiatry and the Sense of Reality*. Oxford: OUP.

Ratcliffe, M., Ruddell, M., & Smith, B. (2014). What is a "sense of foreshortened future"? A phenomenological study of trauma, trust, and time. *Frontiers in Psychology, 5*(1026), 1–11.

Rhodes, J.E., Parrett, N., & Mason, O. (2016). A qualitative study of refugees with psychotic symptoms. *Journal of Psychosis*, 8, 1–11. doi: 10,1080/1 7522439.2015.1045547.

Romme, M.A., & Escher, A.D. (1989). Hearing Voices. *Schizophrenia Bulletin*, 15, 209–216.

Turner, S.W., Bowie, C., Dunn, G., Shapo, L., & Yule, W. (2003). Mental health of Kosovan Albanian refugees in the UK. *British Journal of Psychiatry*, 182, 444–448.

Tribe, R. (2002). Mental health of refugees and asylum-seekers. *Advances in Psychiatric Treatment*, 8, 240–248.

Warman, D.M., Forman, E.V., Henrique, G.R., Brown, G.K., & Beck, A.T. (2004). Suicidality and psychosis: Beyond depression and hopelessness. *Suicide and Life-Threatening Behaviour*, 34(1), 77–86.

5

TRANSFORMATION OF MEANING IN PSYCHOSIS

Are delusions and voices meaningful, and if so, where does such meaning come from and how does it develop? In the following chapter such issues are addressed. First, evidence is presented suggesting that different groups of trauma survivors express distinctive meanings. Next, there is an exploration of how the meaning found in psychotic content, that is, the meaning found in delusions, voices, and psychotic perceptions, is influenced not only by types of trauma but a range of psychological and other processes. To illustrate these diverse contributions to meaning one case is described in depth. Finally, the findings and theories in this chapter are considered in the context of Jaspers's ideas on delusions, in particular, whether we can understand psychotic experiences. It is suggested that a comprehensive open 'cluster' concept of delusions, one that includes a wide range of experiential and other features, may clarify some of these topics.

DOI: 10.4324/9781003044956-5

Comparing the psychotic content and the three types of trauma

In each of the three previous chapters the argument was made that, concerning a specific type of abuse, psychotic content could be found thematically related to the abuse in question. It was striking that participants who had suffered sexual abuse often presented psychotic content that related either to issues of sexuality itself or an idea that voices or attacking others were condemning them. In the chapter on physical abuse it was notable that the majority of participants stated that they thought an attacking other would kill them and in fact do this in a terrible way. The psychotic material presented in the chapter on refugees suggested that the voices, delusional ideas, and perceptions, related either to memories of being attacked by soldiers or others but also sometimes focused on yearning for those who were lost.

Of course there are many other meanings in the changing and evolving psychotic content of the participants which were not related to these themes, and furthermore, there was some crossover of themes, for example, the issue of being seen as a 'paedophile' was present in a participant with physical abuse. There can be themes of sexual activity or violence in any of the three groups but at least by comparative examination of all the cases it was clear that specific themes predominated in the different groups. The psychotic content, however, was not replication of exact details and was clearly subject to various transformations and alterations over time. A great deal of effort in recruiting the participants for this research was specifically to ensure that the physical and sexual abuse groups did not include other types of abuse, that is, the physical abuse had not received sexual abuse and vice versa. To facilitate a direct comparison of the three groups I will present samples which illustrate three types of psychotic content.

Physical abuse

Five of the eight with physical abuse explicitly mentioned extreme violence while one mentioned a lesser form of attack and another thought others saw him as a 'killer'.

> I suddenly thought I'm going to be killed … I thought I was going to be cut up into lots of tiny pieces. (Lesley)

... either kill me, put me in prison, or slowly manipulating my mind. (Greg)

Sexual abuse

The themes relating to sexual abuse were either directly about sexual activity in some way or involved condemnation.

And then the voices were 'She doesn't even feel guilty about what she's done'. ... Where, where you're actually now thinking 'well, if I'm that evil, I must, I must just kill myself now' you know because I can't be evil. (Clare)

I thought that I was a paedophile, and that everybody knew what I was. (Jackie)

Political violence

The themes concerned violence or, in contrast, yearning for those lost.

I hear these voices saying 'Stop, arrest him. Kill him. Kill him'. Like the soldiers used to say in my country. (Frederic)

Concerning his dead mother:

She is telling me 'come join us'. So for me, she came to get me ... they are trying to communicate with me, maybe they are trying to send me a message.

Comparing these diverse statements, from the different groups, suggests that each type of abuse is linked to a psychotic meaning that reflects thematically the specific abuse. The type of abuse has a fundamental and distinctive effect on the sort of meanings found in psychotic experiences. Though such qualitative findings do not yield statistical proof of distribution it seems unlikely that the pattern presented here is mere chance or the product of selective reading. Furthermore, the exposure to abuse continued for years in the early lives of many participants, and the trauma for refugees, though time limited, was extreme and life changing; it is hard to see how such events would not continue to influence the person in profound ways, particularly with regard to meaning.

The many sources of meaning in psychotic content

As stated, the diverse psychotic themes were not exact replicas of the original traumatic events. There was some suggestion in the voices and delusions of those who suffered political violence of some replication of details of events but even here many aspects were clearly thematic transformations. The question therefore arises; what are the diverse sources of psychotic content and what are the psychological and other processes that may be relevant for producing this content? Many sources and processes have been suggested in the literature and here I will present those I believe of most relevance from a psychological point of view (of course there are other processes, such as neurological ones, but these are not covered here).

Emotions and interaction

Looking at the three groups suffering trauma, it is clear that many themes involved negative emotions, attitudes, motivations, and behaviors and that these occurred independently of psychotic experiences. However, if one then compares such themes of emotion, etc., with the content of the psychosis, then parallels are found. Some themes were common across all three groups, in particular, deep mistrust of others and profound problems in establishing social relationships. In the following I will examine how each of the three groups had specific themes.

The participants who had suffered physical abuse were prone to expecting violence or attack in their everyday lives and in situations where psychotic experiences were not occurring. Chris gave an example of expecting attacks in his daily life but he also saw a connection between these expectations and those when he became unwell. He said it was 'frightening being around people' and that 'that people might jump me or something'. He went on to say:

> Like attack me or something, I'd just had this feeling that somebody, the person might just turn on me all of a sudden because, like I said, when you have ideas, when you have incidents that you've seen or that have happened to you in a practical sense, when you become ill, they become the main focus, because I've had that before when someone just jumps me all of a sudden, attack me.

Some of those who had undergone sexual abuse reported a distorted experience of the body and all the participants appeared to be suffering from what might be considered as shame and a sense of degradation, for example, with Hasina:

> They're always looking at, not all of them, but some men look at me in a way that makes me feel dirty.

When asked in what way she answered that she thought others were having 'sexual thoughts'. Here again there is an emotional experience which appears to be common in the life of this person, and comparing this to the ideas given in psychotic content, suggests parallels of meaning in particular concerning condemnation and feeling defective.

For the participants who had suffered political violence one common feature was extreme fear concerning others. Belvie had expressed great fear even about people who happened to be on a bus with her. Togar had felt extreme fear in his country before leaving:

> I used to feel bad like because all the time scared of people, all the times scared about them.

He had to watch out for danger:

> If I, say, meet any violence or fight, I'm gonna die.

And when he got to the UK, for three years he had terrible dreams:

> Like what happened in Sierra Leone, like when they capture, what happened, the terrible things that they was doing you know? So I used to think, I used to get the dreams, wake up and scared dream, you know, the fear.

While some aspects of psychotic content might derive from the trauma itself, alternatively, the above evidence suggests that the types and nature of trauma a person suffers have a long-term influence on a wide range of emotional and social difficulties, and then the latter in turn have an influence upon developing psychotic content.

Motivation

The idea that there may be a connection between meaning in delusions and motivation has a long history, and Jung (1907) presented several case studies as illustration. Rhodes and Jakes (2000) explored how a person's delusions related to motivational themes, that is, concerning what is desired, wanted, or needed, and sometimes, in contrast, what is feared and avoided. A central idea was that the problems, concerns, and related difficulties with needs and goals found in the life of the person would have parallels of meaning manifest in the delusional account. One participant experienced prolonged rejection and intrusive control from her family. In later years she had delusional experiences and hallucinations involving invasive entities such as insects entering her body; her psychotic experience demonstrated her concern and dread that she did not belong with others and that others were attacking her. In contrast, another participant, who was preoccupied with becoming successful as a scientist, had delusions that involved communicating with aliens who would confer upon him special knowledge and power. Isham et al. (2021) noted how grandiose delusions could provide a sense of purpose, identity, or belonging, but having such delusions also brought with them negative consequences, such as the reactions of others.

In Jakes, Rhodes, and Issa (2004) different raters classified independently either delusions or motivational difficulties and found an association between the two. For this study specific motivational themes were generated from interviews with participants, these being: intimacy, love, and sexual relations; achievement and status; social alienation such as not feeling like others or looked down upon; aversion to being controlled by others; and basic fear and dread concerning death, illness, and accidents. The study also developed for each participant a profile of specific delusional themes; this is important since some participants can have combinations of, for example, persecutory and grandiose ideas. Rhodes, Jakes, and Robinson (2005) noted how an individual's delusional account can be complex and have idiosyncratic mixtures of themes.

Which system of motivations might be most useful for understanding delusions is an open question. The possibilities include one such as above, or one derived from an evolutionary perspective such as Gilbert (1989), who suggested attachment, power, belonging to a group, or perhaps an attempted synthesis such as given by Dweck (2017) who delineated three basic needs of predictability, acceptance, competence, and the emergent needs of trust, control, self-esteem or status, and self-coherence. Whatever system is used, it is important we attend to the unique patterns found in the individual.

Biographic details and social context

One obvious source of meaning in the creation of psychotic content is the biography of the person and all the details that are attached to such a history, for example, a person's language, events in the life of the family, the family's specific culture, and the culture of the surrounding society. Harper (2011) describes how a person's social environment, in particular, whether a person feels under various types of social surveillance or threat in relation to social categories such as gender, ethnicity, culture, and class will influence meanings the person holds and which may emerge in psychosis. Rhodes and Jakes (2010) interviewed participants about the onset of delusions; of twenty-three participants, seventeen spontaneously described their delusions as arising in the context of social problems and six described social problems when explicitly ask, with only two not describing any such problems. From the point of view of participants, delusional accounts were focused on social issues. In Harper and Timmons (2021) participants who scored highly on paranoia, but who had no diagnosis, were interviewed concerning their beliefs and how these had been formed. The participants described specific social experiences such as bullying at school, a dangerous neighborhood and family members who expressed distrust.

All such events and processes structure or influence a person and may remain throughout life. Of course, there is no simple relationship of life context and psychotic experience; years ago I was struck by a participant who thought he had become a devil for a period of time, but in fact had always been an atheist and had no interest in religion. Clearly ideas of religion and other major narratives circulating in societies can enter a person's potential repertoire regardless of a person's specific beliefs.

Metaphors and metonymy

In Rhodes and Jakes (2004a) a range of evidence was presented showing how metaphor and metonymy might influence the content of delusions, a topic Jung (1907) explored. One participant when young had noticed a demon representation in a church, and wondered whether she was like such an entity. Years later she was preoccupied with the idea that she was a demon. It is clear that if a person is struggling to understand what is occurring, then that person is likely to make comparisons (following Lakoff, 1987, I will use metaphor and analogy as equivalent), for example, if a person thinks that he or she is being followed, then given the details of a person's experience, the person may begin to think that 'they' are like a drug gang or the Mafia. But such a thought itself creates more fear and the potential for further preoccupation. The claim in the article was not that when someone expresses a delusion or a belief about voices, that the person is intentionally making a metaphorical statement. Rather the claim that the FBI is pursuing a person is meant to be taken literally, that it really is the case. It was therefore suggested that the processes of fusing conceptual domains of meaning (Fauconnier & Turner, 2002), as occurs for a deliberate metaphor, here take place outside consciousness. Some psychotic meaning might be the end product of past conscious comparisons, but some may occur without the person making any deliberate metaphor or comparison. In the end however, by whatever origin, the fusion must occur outside awareness and be delivered in consciousness as something real from the sufferers' point of view (the FBI really are shooting at me).

Chris, who had been physically abused, reported that during a psychotic phase he actively considered if he was 'like one of the disciples'. Lionel, a refugee, reported moments where he might see people in a cafe and noted that 'those people were similar' to the ones he 'saw back home', that is, soldiers who had persecuted him. Comparison between people in the past, associated with violence, and people who might in some way be similar in appearance, seen in the present, are a source of considerable fear in refugees and for others who have suffered different types of assault. One client, reported in Rhodes (2014), had been subjected to domestic violence; she would sometimes become terrified that she had seen the man (who she had left many years before) still on the street and that he might still be following her.

Narration

One source of psychotic content is the person's struggle to understand or narrate what is occurring to them and that the person may re-engage in such struggles to narrate at different moments over long periods of time. An example is given in the case study below. In repeated psychotic breakdowns, often the same or similar content may re-emerge in separate episodes; however, at each occasion it is occurring in a different context and may thus be remembered and rethought in different ways. By repeated narration the very story itself may become distorted and elaborated over time. Such a distortion of narrative was beautifully illustrated in Bartlett (1932) where he told an indigenous American story to participants and then would ask the same individuals to recount the story, sometimes after many years. He found that the story tended to change over time, particularly in the direction of being more compatible with the person's culture and conventions.

The experience of self and other

Abuse is a form of terrible social interaction, whether for a child or for an adult. Such extreme events have a profound impact on how a person goes on to experience the world, upon how memory functions, on ways of interacting, and how the person moves forward with expectations of others. Our memory is a product of learning that we demonstrate in the present and show in our expectations of the future. Theories of memory suggest that some forms of memory may be declarative or implicit, such that we can consciously remember an event or associated meanings, but in contrast some memory systems are non-declarative or implicit and are shown in the exact way we behave. Non-declarative memory includes habits, aversive learning, and instrumental learning, the latter being learning from feedback following actions we take. Squire (2004) and Amodio (2018) argue that there are multiple systems and that they may interact with each other in complex ways depending on the actual relevant activity. A detailed analysis of the relation between trauma, memory and psychosis is given by Moskowitz and Montirosso, (2019) who also note the possible contribution of disturbed and confused communications within a family.

Given the developmental and foundational importance of a person's multiple memories concerning abuse it seems likely that these different sorts of memories provide a basis for experience of others, including relevant meanings, and therefore make a major contribution to the content of psychotic experience.

In analysing interpersonal experience Horowitz (1991) contrasts explicit 'concepts' with 'person schemas' both about the self and the other. Concepts are accessible ideas a person might use in thinking. Person schemas, however, are unconscious and 'summarise past interpersonal experience into integrated, generalised, modular forms'. Person schemas will influence a person's perceptions or feelings directly without awareness of their origin. Concepts and schemas are clearly the produce of experience and memory though may involve other processes such as links to motivation. I will return to this topic in chapter six.

The collapse of everyday certainties

Given that psychotic content can originate in the life experience and psychological processes of a person, the question still arises why the content is so often unusual if not extraordinary and typically violates our deepest expectations of the way the social and physical world operates. For example, a participant who said everyone had a device to transmit messages just about her and that this device was used for nothing else; such a claim implies a perceived world utterly at odds with the one we normally assume (Rhodes & Gipps, 2008). Some delusions even violate the accepted norms of biology and physics, for example, walking through brick walls. In chapter seven I will return to this topic arguing that without grounding in taken-for-granted shared experiences and certainties of the everyday world, that which is given credence by a person will become ever more usual if not impossible.

Case illustration: paranoia and its developmental origin

The many sources and processes, described in the above sections, may over time interact with each other forming psychotic content; in this section I will present one case illustration showing such processes. When I first met William he reported many years of experiencing extreme states of paranoia and attacking voices. He presented as a serious, polite man in his forties who was clearly intelligent and thoughtful. When I first met him he was already at a stage in his life where he was aware of his own difficult history and wanted to discuss some of these often disturbing events. The psychotic meanings of his paranoia and voices, terms he used himself, were complex. In short, his paranoia involved the idea that he had been under threat and constant surveillance by various secret government organisations and terrorist groups. He did not specify the nature of his voices but in general they attacked and insulted him. He reported often feeling anxious, sometimes panic, and for long periods of his life had experienced depression. His diagnosis was of paranoid schizophrenia which he had been given in his early twenties.

He volunteered for the research interview and gave an extensive account of a wide range of experiences including the process of being paranoid and how this had developed over time. He also gave some details concerning the abuse he had received. My aim in this case illustration is to show how the psychotic experiences he underwent acquired meaning in the context of his life history and were further structured by motivational, emotional, and symbolic processes.

Early history

Some facts of his early life are in fact highly distressing and I will only give selective details to illustrate the kind of terrible things that happened. William and his sister had been placed in a home for children at a very young age. He never knew his biological father and reported no specific memories that he could be sure of concerning his mother. After a few years, he and sister were fostered by a couple who ran a farm in an isolated rural area. He said that almost from the beginning he and his sister were subject to repeated beatings and mistreatment. At a very young age, six or seven, he had to do in heavy farm work such as carry bales of straw. He stated:

> I grew up in an atmosphere of impending or threatening violence. I was abused quite strongly with rods, sticks, and verbally, err, err, no love was shown to us.

> It used to be severe slapping around the face and around the behind and legs and the use of a willow rod, stick, thin stick which is very flexible, to use, to beat us around the legs and around the behind. Grabbing tactics, you know, dragging us about, throwing us in to corners, all the sort of heavy handedness, err, and err it was backed up by verbal attacks.

Not only was he abused, but he had to witness the abuse of his sister:

> And my foster mother, I remember to this day, was sniggering and laughing while she was doing it and afterwards. I was upset at the time, I was a year older than my sister, but I knew this couldn't be right, you know.

On this occasion, she was beaten and placed in the dark wearing a sack. If we grow up in a family without such violence, then it is hard to even begin to grasp how this can have occurred and how adults can do such things. The facts above are enough to remind us how extreme abuse can be and to wonder what effect this can have upon children. After many years, he could put up with this mistreatment no longer:

> The two of them attacked me in a room, dragging the clothes off me and I fought back by kicking and I ran off. That was probably the first time I ran away.

On this occasion he thought he could have been killed:

> I realised, I was actually fearful of my life at that time, on that actual episode. I felt that they were capable of killing me.

He returned for some time, and then the beatings stopped; he believed his foster parents were fearful of being reported to social services. He was placed out for short periods to work on other farms and left the area in his early teens.

Memory, experience, and the struggle to understand

My aim, as stated earlier, is to understand the origin of his psychotic content and how it developed. One feature that was very striking was how many comments point to the development of his attempt to understand and narrate. He described the beginning of paranoia:

> But once I reviewed my life with the onset of maturity and so on, I was inclined to dig up aspects of the past and, you know, become paranoid about them, or develop a paranoid attitude about them ... and err, I've more or less been paranoid ever since that, with a major increase in paranoia about seventeen years ago.

Just before this first breakdown, he had written to social services asking for help:

> I wrote a letter to the welfare, around that time in desperation, complaining if you like, that I had problems and err they appeared at my home address around the time I came

home, err, err and just told me 'to pull myself together' that was their entire take on the matter, which was not really helpful, you know?

He added:

I was, I just thought 'well this is more of the same, this is what I'm used to, this is what, I don't expect any more from these people because that's all they're capable of doing'. Err, but err, now I incorporated that into the paranoia at later stages and err, you see my cultural experiences are the main driver in this, in this predicament.

The incorporation was that social services were involved with a terrorist group. He just about coped during his twenties but after a few years he had a breakdown and made a serious suicide attempt. This lead to further developments of his ideas:

It was a continuation by psychologist and psychiatrists and interrogators and police to sort of intimidate me, to coerce me, to control me and though I've gotten away from the worst aspects of that attitude, I still am, inclined to visit it.

This became the 'thread' of meaning discussed in the physical abuse chapter. At its worse, the delusional account now involved the following ideas:

... that people that have controlled me all my life because I was seen as a specimen for manipulation. For, for some time I thought, earlier in the process, some years ago, I thought that err I was actually involved in spying for the secret service when I was about six years of age ... Yeah, yeah and that I was being manipulated so that at a future date they could call me in and say, debrief me, err, I mean that was a very paranoid thing to think.

And given how dangerous these groups really are:

I can develop a scenario where I, I see these people as plotting against me, are ready to kill me.

His paranoid account is an attempt to make sense of his life and suffering. It gives an explanation to why he was placed with people who then abused him. His struggle with understanding, however, started as a child:

> As time progressed, I, I still thought I was doing something wrong somehow but I couldn't really understand what I was doing wrong. I used to fight with myself, you know this must have been wrong, or you know, you must have done this wrong or you're really bad or something.

He added:

> I was in a situation where I was regretful about everything that had happened, not really accepting that I'd been at fault, yet agreeing that I might have been at fault. I don't know if that's a sort of paradox, but err, I was feeling at some level that I was at fault but not really understanding how I was at fault.

His struggle to understand continued right into the present and when his ideas became more paranoid:

> The voices inevitably back up the thoughts with illogical suggestions or rubbish the suggestions and I have to fight those or I have to discuss them in my mind to, to try to get some sort of clarity on the matter to try and make some sense of them. So the voices and the paranoia sort of go hand in hand.

Of course there are many contributions to William's account, but a major one appears to be a fundamental yearning to understand why such terrible things had happened, how to make sense of this, and in addition how to understand new and often difficult experiences occurring as a adult. Delusions are rarely, if ever, simple statements, but rather evolving accounts and narratives that have many aspects and details, all of which can change over time.

What might explain this deep yearning, this motivation to understand? One possibility is that he continued to feel an extreme threat in his daily life and perhaps by understanding 'what was going on' he would be better prepared to deal with it or even to stop the threat. He might also be attempting to fight off a sense of guilt, of worthlessness, of being in the wrong, and to free himself from such feelings. It is also potentially the case that like many who are depressed, he was engaging in a review of personal history to see how he had ended up in such a situation.

A further answer is that even without any conscious awareness of a 'story', his implicit memories would generate terrible feelings in the present, a sort of pre-verbal sense of immanent attack, betrayal, and exploitation, and all these would colour his perceptions and thinking. One might conceived of these feelings as a sort of felt drama or social scenario reoccurring for him in many difficult situations. He was therefore not just thinking in abstract about his life, but already living in a sort of experiential challenge demanding clarification. To engage in deliberate seeking of narrative or explanation, however, did not seem to bring relief, but in fact added to these feelings.

A full answer also requires considering how he was isolated from any shared common knowledge and that as he broke down his fragile coping or hold on living was suspend and feelings of terror, not fully experienced since the time of the abuse, were released. These sorts of processes are covered in chapters six and seven.

The symbolic expression of suffering

Taking the many meanings of his account and comparing these to the events of his life suggests several parallels of meaning or possible connections between different conceptual domains (Lakoff, 1987; Rhodes & Jakes, 2000). The first and major one is that as a child:

I felt that they were capable of killing me

And as an adult:

I see these people as plotting against me, are ready to kill me.

Given the extreme experience of expecting to be killed, that his parents would actually kill him there and then, it seems that this expectation continued into adult life such that others would be seen as similar, that is, they are experienced as lethally dangerous. In a psychotic breakdown, the others who are attacking the adult self are not just similar but are now engaging in actual attempts at murder.

There are other possible metaphorical and the conceptual parallels between different experiential zones. One in particular is that the care staff in the hospital was in fact similar in some key ways to the social services that had originally put him on purpose in a place where he would be abused.

As he proceeded in his life it was always a possibility that caring others, in particular medical and social services, would be seen as similar to those who had mistreated him. Besides the expectation of being killed, there are also similarities in expecting to be mistreated, to be controlled, and to be a 'specimen' for experimentation. His early placement was a sort of abusive experiment and he continued to perceive this in situations as an adult.

Motivations and meaning

It is clear that in his young years a very wide range of needs were violated, in particular the need for safety, love, and respect at the very least. Clearly he was living under such a threat that his very need to stay alive was challenged. His delusional account and psychotic experience expressed this fundamental lack of care and safety and represents or shows how he felt danger in the world. Some delusions might well express what a person wants for example having special knowledge but William had barely ever experienced the basic good things of life such as being loved and feeling safe. His delusional account expresses his fundamental dread of destruction and therefore his need to watch out for attack and to attempt to find some way of being safe.

Contemplating escape

Looking back at his childhood, he thought it likely that he had been depressed and may have gone into some kind of alternative disassociated state. He said that there were moments as a child when he began to contemplate suicide:

> Well, maybe not so much wanting to kill myself but wishing I could lie under the river, those sort of primitive suicidal notions, you know, feeling it would be better you know? That's my opinion yeah, feeling that it would be better and that's approximately where I am now with the suicidal thing.

The symbol of the river here seems to represent some sort of escape: not really dead, but not present in the world in which he suffered and continues to suffer. Also, somehow, that he would be near something natural and peaceful as the flow of a river that suggests movement and life. I have always found this image deeply moving.

An interpretative stance

If a participant such as William says in the context of therapy that he believes the FBI are determined to assassinate him, then in general I believe that we should accept these statements as reflecting the world as experienced for that person. And given the participant is living in such a world we may need to help that person cope with fear and to find ways of feeling safe. Once a person has achieved some calm, stability, and basic self care and expresses an interest in longer term therapy, then it can be useful to think more deeply with the participant what the psychotic content might mean. In the above case study there was an attempt to put the evolving delusional narrative in the context of William's life history, his suffering and motivations. There was also recognition that the delusional content itself might have symbolic or non-literal meanings.

At the core of such attempts at understanding is an interpretive process and this approach first aims to understand what is being said, for example, what exactly does it mean to say the FBI is using surveillance, what is their intention, what kind of entity are they? With more complex meanings one can then think and wonder what sort of issues such an account represents or what sort of experience occurring in everyday life would be similar. In the above it suggested that to feel persecuted by powerful organisations is to feel being under threat as an outsider in society.

When we try to understand another person we are always taking up some sort of interpretive stance, usually without awareness, for example, if someone is expressing how something feels, and uses a metaphor, we know automatically not to take the metaphor at face value. There are perhaps many contexts where we adjust our interpretive stance according to the discursive context and our apprehension of the speaker's intentions. One context might be listening to someone reading a work of fiction. Sometimes we quickly switch from one stance to another, for example, if we switch on the radio expecting the news but then hear a play. There are many types of context requiring diverse interpretative stances such as listening to someone talk while actually asleep, or listening to someone talk who we know has taken powerful hallucinogenic drugs. In all these contexts we adjust automatically how we are to construe what is being said.

I suggest that when we engage in discourse with a person who we think might be suffering from a severe condition such as psychosis, while it is respectful to acknowledge lived experience, it is also useful and respectful to grasp that the person is speaking in the midst of an extreme state, and the person's contact with everyday reality and coping has usually been lost. This I think is respecting the person as that person is now and over time. William in the above case study did not believe his extreme claims most of the time. The issue of whether these were true or false, furthermore, is not a cultural issue. William was fully articulate about the way he moved in and out of the state of paranoia, usually experienced in the context of fluctuating anxiety and depression, and that the state itself was a form of suffering. The psychotic content is not just some alternative and original way of looking at the world. Most people suffering from psychosis and abuse experienced their psychotic content as oppressive and often as horrific.

There can be a danger of imposing our own meanings on what the participant is saying; however, I feel that this can be avoided by cautious investigation of the person's history, motivations, experiences, etc., and respecting the person's perspective on their life and what they've been through. We must also consider our own theories and life experience and how that can influence our reading of meaning. In the end one can only offer alternatives, engage in open dialogue, and accept that it is up to the person whether to consider the feasibility and usefulness of a different perspective.

Are delusions understandable?

It is often claimed that Jaspers (1963) argued that delusions cannot be understood or rather are 'ununderstandable'. By the latter Jaspers did not mean that the actual words or ideas could not be understood; what could not be understood is how the person reached such a judgment or had such a reaction. For example, we readily understand a reaction such as getting upset if a person loses a much cherished object but would find it puzzling if the person became happy. Gipps (2022)Gipps 2022 argues that the critics of Jaspers in general have misrepresented him and that Jaspers was in fact fully aware of the many routes to delusional beliefs. Delusions based on experiences such as hallucinations or depression he called 'secondary'. In contrast, he argued that delusions 'proper' or 'primary' were based on primary delusional experience involving feelings, sensations, and meaning such that we are not able to comprehend how these could occur in the context of what has happened; the experiences or meanings involved seem as if suddenly imposed, having no obvious links with the present situation. They are not understandable in the sense of how one could arrive at that idea from what had been experienced. An alternative term for 'un-understandable' might be 'unjustifiable' in that we cannot understand how the claim is justified or accounted for and we feel baffled. For William, we can understand how he perceives others as dangerous and exploitative, and we might see that the claim of an 'experiment' suggests an analogy, but the leap to believing in a literal 'experiment' as a 'spy' seems unjustified. Hayashi, Igarashi, and Harima (2021) interviewed participants in hospital diagnosed with mainly long-term schizophrenia to investigate primary delusional experiences in the forms of perception, memory, mood, and intuition; they reported that the majority that had had such experiences at some stage. Whether the same would be found for those with other sorts of psychosis, particularly those with abuse histories, was not explored.

I believe Gipps' defense of Jaspers is persuasive. I would, however, wish to note that most delusions as presented in practice appear to be more of a secondary type, that is, they are contextual or experientially derived delusions. Explicit statements concerning pure primary delusional experiences seem rare though are found; for example, in Rhodes and Jakes (2004a) a participant is described who woke up and suddenly knew he had been hypnotised all his life by secret services. The latter sort of delusion tends to have what Rhodes and Jakes (2004b) described as an 'eruptive' nature. They do not however appear to be representative of what most long-term delusions are like most of the time.

I believe that Jaspers selected the feature of 'ununderstandable' concerning primary delusions and relevant experience because he wished to pick out an extremely important and possibly essential element of delusionality (a term suggested by Gipps). The approach of Jaspers, however, appears to me to be too reductive, attempting to cleave all delusions into two clear-cut types: an alternative would be that one accepts an open cluster conception of delusions whereby there are several potential features for specific delusions and different types of delusion. A set of such features, taken together, would be regarded as sufficient to count as a delusion, yet it would be open to debate whether any one particular feature was necessary. Such a conception also allows the comparison of different theories in terms of how they include different or similar features. Gallagher

(2013) developed a cluster or pattern concept of self and this is the approach I am drawing on here.

I wish to suggest that most delusions are in fact complex in content and depend on experience in diverse and complex ways, and furthermore, at least for those delusions that persist, frequently involve an attempt to explain or account for what is going on in the person's world. These are in fact what might be thought of as typical or common delusions whereas expressions of primary delusions based on obvious primary delusional experience are rare, and if occurring, tend to be experienced briefly during a full psychotic breakdown and sometimes in those with the most severe and chronic features of psychosis. I would also suggest that in our everyday conceptions of being deluded there are other accompanying features such as being overwhelmed by perceptions and emotions which have led to various distortions and that the person has somehow lost his or her way. This is the sort of conception found in classical and renaissance literature and which I believe continues in everyday life.

The following is an attempt to construct, from the third perspective, a list of features which could form part of a cluster or pattern conception of delusions. The features have been generated in thinking about the sorts of participants researched in this book, though might apply more widely. A person's state or experiences would be regarded as being delusional to the extent that they matched all or most of these descriptions:

Experiential disturbance and distress

1. The person reports being overwhelmed by experiences felt to be difficult or strange, and which may include a sense that reality has changed.
2. It is shown in diverse ways that the person is in a disturbed and distressed state of mind with regard to perceptions, emotions, and actions, and may suffer anxiety or depression.

Narration and belief

3. There is an attempt to account or narrate or express what is occurring and felt. Over time these claims are intermingled with ongoing related experiences, are inseparable from these, and evolve with mutual influence.

4. There may occur, to varying degrees, all those features typically given in a conventional definition of delusions such as certainty, being false though not necessarily so, being impervious to counterarguments, and not being accepted within the person's cultural tradition or group.

Self, world, and action

5. For the person the world is transformed and something may have been discovered or revealed. The person may act in accordance with these new perceptions and ideas, though sometimes actions seem either inconsistent or their relevance difficult to understand. To those who knew the person when well, he or she now appears changed in fundamental but hard to articulate ways.
6. The claims and relevant experiences, from the outside point of view, imply challenges to the taken for granted everyday shared world and the one usually accepted by the person when not in an altered state.

Justifications and understanding

7. The person argues that something is 'real' which others find difficult or impossible to accept as real. The claims are often unique to the person and are more challenging or puzzling than just error, or ideas found in well-known controversies such as telepathy.
8. There are arguments or justifications given by the person which seem incoherent, puzzling, contain gaps, are hard to follow, and even when clear are not credible or persuasive. Furthermore, the arguments seem to deviate from the way the person may have previously justified claims when well.

Symbolic expression

9. The person would state if asked that they are making literal or factual claims about situations and events; however, there appears to be the use of ideas or images which have their origin in processes of imagination, possibly metaphoric or metonymic thinking. While some figurative expressions might begin in conscious thought, such as making explicit 'as if' comparisons, eventually all claims involve processes which are not deliberate and are outside the person's awareness.

10. The content gives the strong impression or sense of a range of psychological, developmental, and social problems or crises, sometimes including trauma, and may express specific difficulties concerning motivations, emotions, and capacities to relate to others.

Systems of the brain, body, and self

11. There are a range of potential neurological, biological, and psychological alternations, as suggested by diverse theories, and might include changes in cognitive processes, the normal functioning of consciousness, self-awareness, attention, etc.

It might be claimed that the Jaspersian clause eight to some degree is always present for delusions whether or not emerging from primary delusional experience, or based on experiences such as hallucinations, psychotic perceptions, or depressive feelings, but I leave that an open question. A concept such as 'over valued ideas' might only draw on a small number of features, while extreme delusions tend to involve the full range. In contrast, a belief such as alien abduction, while puzzling, does not in fact fit several of the conditions above, for example, the person is usually not disturbed, justifications are given but seem accumulated errors, and similar ideas are encouraged by a sub-culture. It may be that there is no absolute line between delusions and other disturbing and extreme ideas but there are complex overlaps of features between diverse distinctive complex patterns.

Harper (2004) and Bortolotti (2018), in different ways, have argued against any sharp boundary between delusions and other unusual or controversial beliefs; whether there is such a boundary or not, I think we still need to understand what might be, if not unique, then certainly extreme about psychotic beliefs. One answer might well be that delusions tend to satisfy all the conditions above and, in particular, involve factors such as a transformation in a person's relation to the shared world, as will be explored in chapter seven.

Concluding thoughts

Sometimes in textbooks a bold and simple statement is given to summarise a person's psychotic meaning, for example, this man believes he is about to be assassinated by the government. This way of presenting delusions decontextualises the meaning the person has experienced and expressed over time. The more we know, however, about the history, context, and experiences of the person, the more we can begin to understand the meaning, origin, and development of such psychotic content. Our understanding might not be complete, and might profit from a range of further explanatory theories, but that is not dissimilar to our attempts to understand other areas such as dreaming or personality development.

References

Amodio, D.M. (2018). Social Cognition 2.0: An interactive memory systems account. *Trends in Cognitive Sciences, 23*, 21–33.

Bartlett, F.C. (1932). *Remembering*. Cambridge: Cambridge University Press.

Bortolotti, L. (2018). Delusions and three myths of irrational belief. In L. Bortolotti (ed.), *Delusions in context*. London: Palgrave McMillan.

Dweck, C.S. (2017). From needs to goals and representations: Foundations for a unified theory of motivation, personality and development. *Psychological Review, 124*, 689–719.

Fauconnier, G., & Turner, M. (2002). *The way we think: Conceptual blending and the mind's hidden complexities*. New York: Basic Books.

Gallagher, S. (2013). A pattern theory of self. *Frontiers of Human Neuroscience, 7*, 1–7.

Gilbert, P. (1989). *Human nature and suffering*. Hove: Lawrence Erlbaum Associates.

Gipps, R.G.T. (2022). *On Madness*. London: Bloomsbury.

Harper, D. (2004). Delusions and discourse: Moving beyond the constraints of the rationalist paradigm. *Philosophy, Psychiatry and Psychology, 11*, 55–64.

Harper, D.J. (2011) Social inequality and the diagnosis of paranoia. *Health Sociology Review, 20*, 423–436.

Harper, D., & Timmons, C. (2021). How is paranoia experienced in a student population? A qualitative study of students scoring highly on a paranoia measure. *Psychology and Psychotherapy: Theory, Research, and Practice, 94*, 101–118.

Hayashi, N., Igarashi, Y., & Harima, H. (2021) Delusion progression process from the perspective of patients with psychoses: A descriptive study based on the primary delusion concept of Karl Jaspers. *PLoS One*, *16*(4), e0250766. 10.1371/journal.pone.0250766

Horowitz, M.J. (1991). Person schemas. In M. Horowitz (ed.), *Person schemas and maladaptive interpersonal patterns*. (pp. 13–31). Chicago: University of Chicago Press.

Isham, L., Griffith, L., Boylan, A.M., Hicks, A., Wilson, N., Byrne, R. ... Freeman, D. (2021). Understanding, treating, and renaming grandiose delusions: A qualitative study. *Psychology and Psychotherapy: Theory, Research and Practice*, *94*, 119–140.

Jakes, S., Rhodes, J., & Issa, S. (2004). Are the themes of delusional beliefs related to the themes of life-problems and goals? *Journal of Mental Health*, *13*, 619–661.

Jaspers, K. (1963, originally published in 1913). *General Psychopathology* (Transl. J. Hoenig and M. Hamilton), Manchester, UK: Manchester University Press.

Jung, C.G. (1907). The psychology of dementia paecox. *In The Psychogenesis of Mental Disease. Collected Works of Carl Jung, Vol. 3* (1960). London: Routledge and Kegan Paul.

Lakoff, G. (1987). *Women, fire, and dangerous things. What categories reveal about the mind*. Chigaco: University of Chicago Press.

Moskowitz, A., & Montirosso, R. (2019). Childhood experiences and delusions: Trauma, memory and the double bind. In: Moskowitz, A., Dorahy, M.J., & Schäfer, I. (eds.). *Psychosis, trauma and dissociation: Evolving perspectives on severe psychopathology*. (2nd ed.). London: Wiley.

Rhodes, J. (2014). *Narrative CBT: Distinctive features*. Hove: Routledge.

Rhodes, J., & Jakes, S. (2000). Correspondence between delusions and personal goals: A qualitative analysis. *British Journal of Medical Psychology*, *73*, 211–225.

Rhodes, J.E., & Jakes, S. (2004a). The contribution of metaphor and metonymy to delusions. *Psychology and Psychotherapy: Theory, Research, and Practice*, *73*, 211–225.

Rhodes, J.E., & Jakes, S.C. (2004b). Evidence given for delusions during cognitive behaviour therapy. *Clinical Psychology and Psychotherapy*, *11*, 207–218.

Rhodes, J., Jakes, S., & Robinson, J. (2005). A qualitative analysis of delusional content. *Journal of Mental Health*, *14*, 383–398.

Rhodes, J.E., & Jakes, S. (2010). Perspectives on the onset of delusions. *Clinical Psychology and Psychotherapy, 17*(2), 136–146.

Rhodes, J., & Gipps, R. (2008). Delusions, certainty, and the background. *Philosophy, Psychiatry, and Psychology, 15,* 295–310.

Squire, L.R. (2004). Memory systems of the brain: A brief history and current perspective. *Neurobiology of Learning and Memory, 82,* 171– 177.

6

PSYCHOSIS AND THE FRAGMENTED SELF

The transformation and fragmentation of the self, it will be argued, are key features for those who have experienced trauma and psychosis. In this chapter illustrations and analyses are given of the diverse states or parts of the self and how these might contribute to the psychotic experience of self and other. One section considers how hallucinations are generated by a fearful part of the self holding memories formed during abuse. Finally there is a discussion of how a person's coping lived or enacted identity may be lost during the experience of depression for those with psychosis.

States of the self

Many therapists and theorists have now suggested that we can view the self as composed of several different states or ways of being. A person might be aware that they have different manifestations of their personality, for example, typically competent but sometimes highly indecisive. However, it can also be the case that there are parts of the self, such as extreme distress

DOI: 10.4324/9781003044956-6

or anger, which manifest themselves rarely and of which the person is hardly aware, if at all. To what extent diverse parts are separated from each other, and what these different parts might be, has been the focus of many theories. Rowan (2010) presents a detailed historical review of these conceptualisations and therapies. Given there are so many theories, Rowan suggests that perhaps we should see all these typologies as diverse possible 'personifications' of the self and that there can be no one definitive classification. I will return to this topic in chapter eight.

The concept of complex states of the self became apparent in the themes presented in the chapters on sexual and physical abuse, for example, to engage in 'self-attack' or 'self-degradation'. In the analysis of these and other themes it was suggested that the concept of self state may be useful in understanding the experience of those with psychosis and abuse and might also be useful in therapy. This chapter collects together those ideas and presents further analysis.

How are states of the self defined? There are, as stated, many different definitions with varying emphases. For this chapter I have used the following definition: a state of the self is a pattern of emotions, thoughts, behaviours, and attitudes which manifests itself as interconnected; furthermore, it is an open pattern, such that it repeats itself over time and yet might also change some of its constituents. This definition tries to capture how we might say a person can have different 'sides' or that 'sometimes he is like a different person'. This is the concept that I have used to re-analyse the interviews for this chapter. This conception is therefore broader than the one given by van der Hart, Niejenhuis, and Steele (2006) who focus on states produced by trauma, that is, dissociated states (discussed later).

Common self states in psychosis and trauma

What are the different experiential states of the person found to be common in the three groups and which can occur outside the context of the symptoms of psychosis or depression? For example, a person might hear intermittent voices but also experience a state of extreme fear, with or without the voice occurring. I will first focus on the participants with physical and sexual abuse and summarise the findings for refugees separately. Five states of self were very common: destabilising anger, dread of others, self critical attack, feeling inferior and/or defective, and feeling isolated. Two other states, one concerned with control, and one of being withdrawn, were also present but less common.

Destabilising rage

Of the fifteen participants who experienced child abuse fourteen expressed strong states of feeling anger or rage. Rita (CPA) stated:

> I tremble and I shake with temper. It's just not a very nice experience. I don't hit out or anything like that, it's just not a very nice experience.

In another part of the interview in discussing relationships she added:

> Err, anger…I'm angry at myself and others.

Here anger becomes an overwhelming experience and has negative effects on keeping a relationship. She shakes as if she is about to come apart and the experience is felt through and in her body.

Sue (CSA) stated:

> Even now if I, if I read about something, if even read about somebody in the news being raped or something, instantly I feel like smashing my head against the wall or something like that.

And if the man was present, then:

> If I was around, if I was around the woman and the man, I probably would attack him.

Sometimes the extreme state of rage is expressed during a breakdown. The episode described here by Peter (CPA) followed a long period of feeling the neighbours were making noises on purpose.

> Now the people upstairs when, when I, when I lost it, when I flipped out two years ago umm, I came back and I was shouting a lot, smashed the flat up, smashed the room, shouting and that sort of stuff, wasn't in control of myself at all, umm, in saying that I never wanted to hurt or harm anyone, and that was the other point, you see I'd go out and get pretty wound up by people by what they were doing outside and I'd come back to my place and have it out in my space.

Sally (CPA) was very aware how anger actually had effects on her personality:

> It's making me into somebody that I'm not, it's not like my personality to be like this and I don't like it.

Here we see how she is aware of one version of her personality but that there was also another version, the self in anger, which she saw as 'not' her. Clearly her anger is extreme and potentially dangerous.

The topic of abuse or rape for Jackie (CSA) was highly disturbing; she described her reaction after the rape of her daughter:

> Yeh, I mean, at first I wanted to go out and kill the bloke who'd done it. I couldn't sleep I was so angry. In fact I was walking around late at night with a knife in my hand looking for him, and things like that.

From the interviews alone, it is not possible to say whether these states of anger are in some way replications of the anger of that person as a child, that is, the concept expressed in Young et al. (2003). The states are extreme, affecting or changing personality, and sometimes seem linked by meaning to past trauma themes. There is a sense with some participants of the anger overwhelming them, of destabilising the coherence of self and its ability to act in a practical way.

Dread of others

States of fear were very common with only one participant not explicitly mentioning it. Most often the fear concerned other people, as for Rita (CPA):

> Anything, meeting people, I was afraid of other people actually... oh gosh, I thought I might make them angry, I didn't want to make them angry... just in case they lash out or attacked me.

Here we see not only fear but a concern that others might be violent and this seems to reflect her experience of physical abuse. William (CPA) had many social fears but also fears concerning a wide range of topics:

I have severe anxieties, umm. These are usually centered around my future, my present, my prospects …these are stress points and I can, if I allow myself, I can get extremely anxious, I mean totally agitated, twitching umm, hyperventilating.

Here fear or anxiety seems to become more extreme, perhaps involving aspects of panic; again, the body is affected. Clare (CSA) gave:

Well, you have a lot of fear. I would have a lot of fear in that situation umm, and I'd be questioning the way I was reacting to what was being said.

Zoe (CSA) stated:

I'm frightened at night sometimes just to go to sleep. I take my medication but I'm frightened someone's gonna get in my flat. That's what I'm frightened of. And I put things up against the door, wedge it between the lock and the banisters. You know, sort of thinking someone might come in and assault me. But umm, then I try and logicalize it, and I think 'is it possible, if they get through my roof, if they get through my door'? and I sort of check, I do that during the day as well.

It is possible that this fear relates to experiences Zoe had as a child of someone entering her room. Toni (CSA) was afraid of losing her memory. She had mentioned writing and when asked what sort replied:

Well anything and everything that springs to mind. Coz, oh yeh, I have a fear of losing my mind…well I'm afraid of getting amnesia.

She said this started in her late teens. It is possible that Toni was concerned about losing her memory in general, since she was afraid of losing the memories of what had happened to her during abuse. Participants could have fear about many topics, but the most common concerned other people and in some instances there was a possible thematic link to early trauma.

Feeling defective and attacking the self

In chapters two and three, the themes of feeling oneself to be defective, inferior, or bad were described as combined with the theme of attacking oneself, in particular, to be extremely critical; the two often go together.

However, comparing all the cases, from all the groups, it is clear that sometimes the two themes are experienced as separate; that is, for some participants there could just be a feeling of being defective, with or without conspicuous self criticism. Examples of a profound sense of feeling incompetent were expressed by Chris (CPA):

> Well, because I feel incompetent it just affects everything basically. It affects me getting up in the morning and doing anything for myself, it affects me having a conversation with somebody ...It affects me wanting to study anything, anything in particular now, yeah.

Clearly this state is very pervasive for Chris and seems to extend into many areas. Another example came from Irene (CSA):

> I'm feeling redundant and quite useless.

The feeling and state of being defective, however, can also explicitly touch how the person relates to others, as described by Lesley (CPA):

> So I felt really sort of like, no one, why would anyone like me, why would anyone want to be my friend, you know, I just felt so sort of insecure that I sort of depended on people I didn't even really like sort of thing, because I felt like it was, I had such low self worth.

Several examples of self-attack were given in earlier chapters. Another example was given by Hasina (CSA):

> Oh, not again, or why have you got to put yourself through this? Or, you're so stupid, you know.

While self-attack might augment a person's sense of failing, or feeling somehow defective, it does seem that this sense or feeling of being defective might exist independently and have developed in early years.

Seeking control

Seven of the participants described issues concerning 'control', discussed here by Rita (CPA):

When I'm meeting new people, yes, and sometimes if I'm unsure of a situation, like I have to be in control, I very much have to be in control, I don't like things getting out of control … and my anxieties can just get out of control or feel like they are out of control or other people can get out of control.

Perhaps 'control' means several things: above it seems to be about what may happen in a social context, about self, and about what others might do. She also needs to keep her feelings under control. It is not specified what might happen if not controlled; however, it does seem to indicate danger. Jackie (CSA) had been aiming to get more control over years:

I'm feeling more in control of myself. Looking over the years now, I feel more in control. But I still feel pretty down and depressed, but I do feel more in control nowadays than I did years ago. Feel like I'm getting my own life back a little bit.

She gives having control great value even if she is still depressed. She is getting her life back which contrasts with somehow not having her life before. Control seems to be seen by participants as a way of having a better life, stopping danger, and a way of coping.

Becoming withdrawn

Five of the participants mentioned what appeared to be a deliberate strategy to keep a distance between themselves and others. Sally (CPA) stated:

You know, to be quite reserved is quite a good thing.

And Zoe (CSA):

I find members of the public very difficult to deal with. I find people are very aggressive very judgemental you know? And I sometimes just want to withdraw from people.

Toni (CSA) stated:

I can't express my anger. I have to keep my anger under control.

And added:

But I try, avoid, not to cry, just to get, just so they can't gloat

Toni expects difficulties and that others will enjoy mistreating her. Some participants suggested that withdrawing had started in childhood. Sue (CSA) said of herself as a child:

That made me sort of like withdraw, and sort of like withdraw into myself, like I was the only one in this world.

To withdraw here seems to be a sort of protection. Some part or aspect of herself is put within herself, as if she could hide in a place where she is the only one and what appears to others is not the self that can be hurt. If one is in oneself, then the person is not with others. What the person has withdrawn is not obvious, but perhaps connection, talk, or actions with others.

Lonely isolation

All participants with physical abuse and six with sexual abuse described a profound sense of being not connected to others. I will not give extensive details here since these are given in chapters two and three. The theme in the physical abuse chapter concerned 'damaged intimacy'; the person felt it very difficult to have relationships and often this was due to issues of anger. For those with sexual abuse the theme was called 'a sense of being different'; these participants also felt great distance from others, had enormous problems with relationships, and tended to emphasise a specific theme of feeling different to others. Several talked about specific difficulties of sexual relationships. Some participants noted that their difficulties had started in childhood, as Rita (CPA):

Difficulties in relationships I suppose, I haven't had many relationships. I think a lot of what happened to me as a child came out in my relationships.

The common theme, as stated, was having profound social problems with potential friends, people in general, and intimate partners; there was a pervasive and strong sense of being isolated and often feeling lonely.

Refugees

All seven refugees expressed profound states of fear; in contrast to the groups suffering child abuse, only one refugee mentioned anger. There was also no specific mention of themes such as attacking the self, seeking control, or feeling defective. A state of being distressed was mentioned by all seven that included crying, feelings of misery, and sadness, and one mentioned a pain in the 'heart'. The refugees often commented on missing those from the past, but this was not presented as a specific or long-term problem of the ability to connect to others.

Overview of states of self

For the participants who had suffered child abuse the diverse states of self were destabilising rage, dread of others, self-attacking criticism, feeling defective, being isolated, being withdrawn, and seeking control. Such states are not unique to those with psychosis and abuse and might be found with or without other conditions, though sometimes in a milder form. The states presented here overlap with, though are not exactly the same, as the sorts of states described by Young et al. (2003) or Fisher (2017), both discussed in chapter eight. Given that the participants were asked questions that did not assume any particular type of self state then these questions may reveal the states that are most common and familiar to the participants. I believe it is likely, however, that if these participants were given formal questionnaires, or extended interviews in a clinical context, then other states of self would also be revealed.

Psychotic identity states of self and the perceived other

In the interviews with those who had survived abuse it was conspicuous that some reported a time during psychosis when they had been transformed in a profound way, for example, one had become a 'disciple'. It was suggested that the identity of being a disciple might be the produce of a psychotic transformation of a state or part of self, in this case, one of feeling vulnerable to attack. The person had moved from 'I feel attacked yet am innocent' to 'I am a persecuted disciple'. Several theorists have explored the idea that having disturbed parts of the self might contribute to psychosis (see later section). In this section I wish to examine how psychotic experience might well be understood as a transformation of states of the self such that new 'identities' are created. Here 'identity' might include, for example, age, sex, roles in society, types of status, and certain types of ability, but would not include changing emotional states of self or personality.

Psychotic transformations of parts of the self

Analysing the interviews suggested three different psychotic types of identity; for each type I will suggest possible non-psychotic states of self that may have contributed to the psychotic identity state.

The psychotic terror identity

Chris (CPA) for a period of time considered himself to be an actual disciple of Christ who was being persecuted. Greg (CPA) thought of himself at one point as 'adopted' and that his parents were about to kill him. William described being a 'specimen' for experimentation: this suggests someone with no power of choice, who has to just suffer whatever happens at the hands of the experimenters, however terrible, and which leaves him completely vulnerable. This appears parallel to what he did in fact experience over many years of abuse and neglect, as described in chapter five. At one time he also thought that perhaps as a child he had been sent as a 'spy' into the family that adopted him; this appears to underline a sense of being an outsider. Given a person carries a strong sense of being vulnerable, of being in danger, and furthermore, that this feeling of vulnerability was experienced as a young child, then it seems possible that as such a person undergoes psychosis, then this state of vulnerability is expressed as a new psychotic identity.

The psychotic power identity

Some participants suggested that they had experienced feelings of being strong and powerful during psychosis. Peter had considered himself to be 'Jupiter' for a short period of time and Lesley had believed that she had magical powers. Chris believed that he was extremely rich and that others knew but would not say or admit this. It seems possible that such transformations involve wanting to be powerful or engaging in fantasies of power.

The psychotic terrible identity

Greg (CPA) had during psychosis come to believe that he was a 'killer'. Jackie (CSA) came to believe that, in the media and by the public, she was known to be a 'paedophile' and for a time that she believed that she had killed her father. Peter (CPA) also thought that perhaps he was a 'killer' and was concerned that others saw him as a 'monster'.

Perhaps such identities mainly express a feeling of being defective; however, for some, feeling defective is also mixed with a sense of being powerful. Feeling oneself to be such a terrible individual or entity could also be in itself a source of fear given the imagined responses of others who might condemn or attack.

Summary of psychotic identity states

The above analyses suggested parallels between psychotic identities and emotional and relational self states. A central argument is that the multiple emotional and relational states of the person may provide a sort of content, meaning, or set of dispositions which are transformed into psychotic experience. It seems possible that a major contribution to psychotic terror identity was the non-psychotic self state of the dread of others. The non-psychotic feelings of being defective may have contributed to the psychotic identity of being terrible or bad.

How states are transformed will involve a multitude of processes, some involving meaning and other psychological processes as in chapter five, and some involving the capacity to maintain a sense of the real versus unreal or imaginary, as will be discussed in chapter seven. Other potential processes would also include some of those outlined in chapter one.

Psychotic perception of the other

In the midst of psychosis there was often a strong sense of persecution by various types of persons or entities that engaged in attacking the self. I wish to hypothesise that these perceived external entities are the product of remembered but transformed images of the person or persons who were abusive. The interviews suggested two broad categories of attacking other.

The attacking quasi-human entity

Some participants experienced persecution by a non-human entity or quasi-human entity. Mirza (CPA) and Lesley (CSA) both spoke of a 'demon'. Hasina believed herself to be persecuted by 'spirits' which formed part of a curse upon her mother and then herself. In chapter nine there is an example of a physically abused person who experienced a terrible devil's voice; when asked to imagine this voice she gave the image of a fist. There were powerful thematic parallels between her present psychotic experience and past emotional and physical abuse. Perhaps for some participants the memories are so terrible that only something quasi-human, a thing or a sort of 'it', can express the person's deepest dreads.

The attacking 'they'

The most common attacking entity, experienced by twelve participants, was an unspecified 'they'. One version of this is the situation where at different times it is a different person or persons who are spying or at-tacking, but these all individuals come from one collective such as the FBI. A second version is when the participants are in a specific social situation surrounded by others, for example, in a cafe where a number of in-dividuals are perceived to have ideas of contempt or violence. For Zoe and Sue (both CSA), others in public made insulting comments concerning sexual activity. For Toni (CSA), the others she encountered were not only insulting but posed a threat of further sexual abuse. For Chris (CPA) un-specified others were potentially plotting his death. As described, William (CPA) was the target of malignant terrorist and professional groups who sent their members to carrying out actions against him.

Benign transformations of self and other

Both Chris and Greg (both CPA) also described how in a time of psychotic breakdown they felt and believed themselves to be actual children again.

During these transformations they did not, however, report a state of fear; the experiences in fact seem to be compensatory, as if expressing a desire for safety or to be cared for, that is, something they rarely had as children. Irene encountered the spirit of her dead grandfather who had come to ask for forgiveness, that is, the very man who sexually abused her. Several of the refugees reported seeing or hearing lost relatives call out to them and these were usually seen as comforting figures.

Summary of psychotic self and other identities

In the above analyses there was an attempt to compare psychotic identities states with the earlier emotional and relational self states reported in the interviews. A central argument is that the emotional and relational states of the person may provide a sort of content or meaning, which is then transformed by psychotic experience.

Twelve participants experienced some sort of attacking 'they' and three a quasi-human entity; of these, eight underwent this experience from the position of their usual non-psychotic selves, while for the other seven there was sometimes the experience of being under attack from the 'they' but at the same time the identity of the participant was transformed by psychosis, for example, into a 'disciple'. Of the eight with no psychotic identity change, five experienced an attacking 'they' and three an attacking quasi-human entity. In sum, just less than half had the experience of a psychotic identity and perceived psychotic other, while just over half of the participants had only a psychotic attacking other.

An experience of persecuting psychotic others, that is, the 'they' or quasi-human entity, might find their origin in several sources; one might be that the terrified vulnerable part of self carries with it an image or memory (declarative or non-declarative) of that which was attacking and terrible during the experience of child abuse. Destabilising rage might also suggest the image of another person who is attacking. Likewise, feeling inferior or defective implies the others who are perceived as superior and condescending.

It is likely that many aspects of child abuse were either forgotten or dissociated (Van der Hart, Niejenhuis, & Steele, 2006) by the participants and that these usually inaccessible memories, later during psychosis, manifested themselves in the perception of the 'they' or quasi-human entity. The various types of memory, including those that may be dissociated, might all contribute in their different ways to the production of terrible psychotic imagination.

In trying to understand psychosis we perhaps need to conceptualise that for an individual there is an experiential and imagined self-other pair and how one or both of the pair may undergo psychotic transformations that reproduce experiences of child abuse. The attacking other might somehow be based on the original abusers or might involve a sense of how the participants imagined disapproving 'others' in general.

Hallucination as other person-schemas of the vulnerable self

Given a terrified part of the self might have person schemas of an attacking other, then it is possible that when a person has a hallucination of an attacking voice then the voice, or vision, has its origin in the person schema. The other person schema is such that it can generate feelings of attack and make the person prone to expecting danger. Benign voices might also emanate from schemas of the other but in this case schemas of caring others that the person might have experienced or wished to experience. Some of those who have been abused will have experienced caring treatment at least sometimes as well as mistreatment.

Horowitz (1992) also considers how self and other schemas may operate with 'scripts', that is, expectations about how an interaction might unfold with another person. For example, given the experience of a feeling of being approached, then one might expect an attack to follow. The activated 'live' schemas here will form the basis of expected social exchanges from which the attacking voices are created.

A further point about schemas, as discussed by Young et al., is that any experience generated by them is automatically taken for 'real' by the person and the experiences can be thought of as involving a sort of 'conviction' demonstrated in reactions. Following this analysis, then the origin of voices might actually originate in convictions and meanings held by the person and is not an error in the perceptual system, the latter theory on voices being put forward by Janet (Moskowitz & Heim, 2011). Hallucinations will therefore be a variant of believing something so much that we imagine it and even perceive it. An additional and essential point is that such experiences, and relevant schemas, may be held by parts of the self.

Ratcliffe (2017) speculates on the role of fearful anticipation and considers how the anticipation of one's own thoughts might contribute to an experience of such thoughts as being more like perception or as not coming from the self. I wish to borrow from Ratcliffe's ideas concerning anticipation but in the following way: at a time of distress the person feels disturbed and has a sense of threat, though why or how is often not known to the person. As described in chapter five, the participants were greatly preoccupied with threats in their everyday lives and ones that occurred independently of psychotic symptoms. These thoughts or fearful anticipations themselves can further activate the inaccessible vulnerable and distressed states which then generate, through the triggering of relevant dispositions, the creation of perceptions of external entities. Given an initial experience of a voice the person enters into yet more fear and more anticipation about what they are about to experience.

To recap, the central points are: 1) traumas create dispositional schemas concerning attacking entities; 2) the schemas are held by a vulnerable or child part to which the adult self normally has little or no access; 3) during a breakdown the vulnerable parts of the self are strongly activated and generate feelings and expectations not under control of the everyday adult self and which feel as if they are not generated by the self but come from elsewhere or from a different agent. Of course, all these processes intermingle with other processes, contributing to psychosis and amplify each other.

Psychosis and parts of the self: a brief history

The idea that psychosis might involve fragmented or dissociated parts of the self has a long history. The idea was discussed in the nineteenth century by several writers but Janet in particular developed the idea that the self fragments in response to trauma and he coined the term 'dissociation'. The idea of dissociation was then used by Bleuler and Jung to conceptualise schizophrenia in particular which they differentiated from psychosis. Moskowitz and Heim (2011) argue that Bleuler has often been misrepresented and that his core argument is that schizophrenia involves fragmentation and separation of personality functions in a similar way to the processes described by Janet concerning dissociation. On several occasions Bleuler used the word dissociation but eventually he developed and settled for the new term of 'schizophrenia'. Considering the arguments given by Moskowitz and Heim, it seems likely that Bleuler was the first to put forward the idea that schizophrenia involves parts of the self.

Bleuler wrote in 1905 (quoted in Moskowitz & Heim, 2011): 'independently of the conscious personality, wishes and fears regulate ideas to their liking and combine them in a compact complex, whose expressions emerge as "hallucinations"; these appear to be so consequential and deliberate that they simulate third person... But it is merely a piece of the split off personality; it represents aspirations of this personality which would otherwise be suppressed'. Although Bleuler usually argued that this process of 'splitting' involved physical processes, Moskowitz and Heim show that that Bleuler did in fact consider the possibility that these changes could be initiated psychologically (Moskowitz & Heims, 2011). Jung was also much influenced by the ideas of Janet but Jung greatly extended the conception of parts of the self to include ones that were not the produce of trauma. Janet's main work was not on psychosis, but he did write several papers on the topic (reviewed in Moskowitz, 2008) and in 1947 suggested that hallucinations related to 'delusional paranoia' involved 'a fragmentation of the conscious personality' (quoted in Moskowitz et al., 2019, p. 140).

The notion that psychosis involved a disintegration of parts of the self was employed in diverse ways in the following decades. The concept occurs in Berne (1961), who had been influenced by Federn (1952); Berne argues that 'childhood ego states exist as relics in the grown-up and that under certain circumstances they can be revived' (p. 30). He presents three main types of ego state, namely child, adult, and parent, and states that in psychosis the child state is experienced as the 'real self' and the adult self is 'decommissioned' (p. 139). He gives an example of a woman who heard an aggressive voice, speaking like her father when intoxicated and using the same sort of extreme language. Laing (1960) spoke of a divided self where the person presents a false self to the world and this was seen as developing in the context of difficult family relationships.

More recently, for trauma in general, the structural dissociation model (SDM) has been developed by van der Hart et al. (2006); it explicitly builds on the original ideas of Janet but also draws on other writers on trauma such Myers (1940). The SDM argues that after trauma a person may present what they term an 'apparently normal personality' (ANP) but on other occasions there are manifest highly disturbed emotional states of personality (EPs). The ANP and EP, in this theory, both have difficulties such as restricted fields of consciousness and in general less ability and energy to integrate experience. In the SDM the emotional parts of the personality are related to basic biological and motivational systems such as fight, flight, and freezing.

The idea that parts of the self are important in psychosis is also discussed by Van der Hart, Niejenhuis, and Steele (2006) in the form of 'dissociative psychosis', where psychotic features such as a voice are generated by the emotional parts of the self. Moskowitz and Corstens (2007) present research arguing that voices are dissociative and outline a therapy where voices are interviewed to explore their history and purpose. Related concepts have been used by Longden et al. (2012) using a dissociative model of voices. Ideas of the fragmented self in psychosis will be further discussed in chapters seven and eight.

Sass and Parnas (2003) also discuss the self with regard to schizophrenia; their approach, however, is quite different in that the main focus is not on the sorts of emotional or attitudinal states discussed in this chapter but rather features such as 'exaggerated self-consciousness' or a 'weakened sense of existing' as a source of awareness and action. It is an interesting question as to what extent this might overlap or not with the states of self describe earlier, but cannot be explored here.

Depression and the destruction of lived identity

In the group of refugees, the majority expressed sometimes overwhelming feelings of distress and that they felt depressed. Several also mentioned that in some fundamental way they were no longer the same person or self. One stated that he was a 'broken self'. Unlike the participants abused in childhood, the traumatised refugees could remember the time before trauma when they had lived well and were aware that their sense of self had changed. There was a similar finding of an altered sense of self in research looking at reactive and chronic depression without psychosis (Rhodes, Hackney, & Smith, 2019; Smith & Rhodes, 2015). I wish to explore what this loss of self might involve and will draw upon theory concerning depression and the self.

Although a range of diverse descriptions were used by the refugees, and the participants in the depression research, these all seemed to suggest a change in an aspect of their normal selves. Gallagher (2013) presented a list of possible features of the self and this included the experience of being a minimal self, awareness of body and space, basic capacities to relate and interact with others, emotions, cognitive abilities, the capacity to narrate one's life history, and extended aspects of self, such as one's clothes, a home, and situated aspects such as cultural practices and the environment. From the interviews there was no obvious evidence to suggest that such fundamental features or capacities of the person did not continue, although sometimes they might be severely altered. The question therefore arises; if the 'self' is broken or lost, yet the sorts of fundamental features listed here continue, what exactly has changed or been suspended?

Given the findings above, and drawing on certain concepts from psychology and phenomenology, I wish to argue that what has altered is the person's former coping and functioning 'identity' and directly linked to that is the loss of a person's capacity to realise in everyday actions a conception of their identity and the motivation to instantiate or create that identity. Drawing on Heidegger (1927) and arguments given by Blattner (2006), I will argue that a person not only might have ideas and aspirations for the future but also that these motivations to live and exist in a certain way are manifest in everyday actions and reactions; for example, if someone wishes to be a teacher, then that person will engage in a multitude of small actions, such as preparing lessons, presenting oneself in a certain way in front of a class, but also longer term complex actions such as training. With this put-into-action identity will come a whole set of commitments and values shown in the smallest details of a person's life. This making concrete of a way of being can be thought of as a person's lived or enacted identity and one that is created in the context of relations with others and surrounding society. Our identity is not just what we think we are or say, but what we do and how we react and feel over long periods of time. This lived identity clearly involves not only aiming for something in the future but to realise, in the present, a way of living.

A feature of depression is that it strikes at the very core of our hopes, desires, motivations, and capacities to live in a specific way in a certain context. A person who has as central to their identity that of being a teacher, and loses this purpose and way of living, may then feel completely lost and cannot replace the former identity. At such times Rhodes et al. (2019) presented evidence from in-depth interviews suggesting that the person will experience periodic agonising engulfment (involving feelings of sinking, being enclosed in darkness, with accelerating negative ideas such as despair and convictions of destruction) but also will feel protracted emptiness and an experience of no longer being their former selves, in fact of losing their lived identity. To the extent that a person's lived identify involves commitment to others such as being a partner or parent, then such loss also profoundly changes how a person relates to others and how it feels to relate to others. The loss of others was very striking in the interviews with refugees.

An additional point concerning lived identity is that this involves not just specific actions but habits and ways of doing things repeated over time; Husserl (Moran, 2014) spoke of the 'ego style' as involving a 'habitus', that is, a way or manner of being and doing acquired over time. As a person becomes ever more accustomed to being a teacher or a partner in a relationship, these habits realised in the everyday world become more automatic, and if there is an abrupt change, such that they can no longer be used or manifest, then the person will feel something core is lost. It is also of course the case that the particular ways of being, or habits of a person, occur within a culture and the latter provides a potential repertoire of ways of being which are realised by the specific individual in a specific context. The fact that refugees found themselves in a very different culture, where developing new roles and ways of interacting was difficult, might itself have added further challenges.

All the refugees experienced extraordinary changes in their life which involved witnessing violence, unexpected death and loss, and then the flight to another country. They subsequently experienced a wide range of social and mental difficulties, and as stated, were often depressed. As a consequence, their former pre-trauma coping lived identities were brushed aside or in fact destroyed by these events. If we also accept the theory that any person will have different parts or states of self, then it may be that for these participants their former coping adult self, that is, the very one that constituted their usually functioning lived identity, had been lost and other parts, for example, a part which feels desperate and vulnerable was released. A process such as torture is in itself likely to create a terrified part of self. The person, having lost their pre-trauma identity, might then go on to develop a sort of 'apparently normal part of the personality' (ANP), as described by Van der Hart, Niejenhuis, and Steele (2006) or what Fisher (2017) called the 'going on with normal life' self which just about manages; the interviews suggested that this too periodically breaks down and I believe was central to the continuous suffering of the refugees.

To recap; to understand the developmental trajectory of refugees we need to use the three concepts of a pre-trauma functioning lived identity, and then after trauma, the two parts of self, that is, an ANP and the EP. Once an ANP is sufficiently developed and functions in the everyday world, then this might keep at bay the extremities of depression; however, all too often the ANP is fragile, periodically breaks down, and opens up the possibility of being dominated by terrified states of self and deeper depression.

Turning to the comments by those with child abuse it is clear that practically all the participants reported severe depression over many years, usually beginning in childhood. It would appear that at least for some there had been a period of managing in the everyday world, for example, both Mirza and William worked for short periods of time. It is not clear, however, that at such times the participants were free from difficulties such as anxiety and feeling profoundly different from others. Rather, again using the SDM, the self that managed to find employment was the fragile ANP, or as Fisher says, the 'going on with normal life' self. With the onset of psychosis, or in periods when psychosis becomes more powerful, it might be that the parts of the self, described in the earlier sections such as the self in terror or rage, come to be predominant for the person. The way such parts of the self might be disconnected from a grounded sense of the everyday world is a topic I will turn to in the next chapter.

Concluding comments

In this chapter several common states of self experienced by the participants were described: destabilising rage, dread of others, self-attack, feeling defective, and seeking control and withdrawal. It was then suggested that aspects of these might become transformed during psychosis such that a state of feeling terror is transformed into to new psychotic identity. Hallucinations were conceptualised as the product of other person schemas held by terrified child parts of the self. The theory was then presented that for traumatised adults who also experience depression, not only has the old pre-trauma functioning lived identity been destroyed, but the new post-trauma just-about-coping self, that is, the self just about keeping its contact with and in the everyday world, might be periodically suspended, allowing other extreme parts to emerge and predominate. I will return to the topic of states of self and trauma in the next chapter and explore how this feature might be an important contribution to psychosis. The topic of states of self will also be featured centrally in the chapters on therapy.

References

Berne, E. (1961). *Transactional analysis in psychotherapy*. New York: Grove Press.

Blattner, W. (2006). *Heidegger's being and time*. London: Bloomsbury Academic.

Federn, P. (1952). *Ego psychology and the psychoses*. New York: Basic Books.

Fisher, J. (2017). *Healing the fragmented selves of trauma survivors*. New York: Routledge.

Gallagher, S. (2013). A pattern theory of self. *Frontiers of Human Neuroscience*, 7, 1–7.

Heidegger, M. (1927/1962). *Being and time* (Transl. Macquarrie, J. & Robinson, E.). Oxford: Blackwell.

Horowitz, M.J. (1992). Person schemas. In M. Horowitz (ed.), *Person schemas and maladaptive interpersonal patterns*. Chicago: UCP.

Laing, R.D. (1960). *The divided self*. London: Tavistock Publications.

Longden, E., Madill, A., & Waterman, M. (2012). Dissociation, trauma, and the role of lived experience: Towards a new conceptualization of voice hearing. *Psychological Bulletin*, 138, 28–76.

Moran, D. (2014). Edmund Husserl's phenomenology of the habitual self. *Phenomenology and Mind*, 6, 26–47.

Moskowitz, A., & Corstens, D. (2007). Auditory hallucinations: Psychotic symptom or dissociative experience? *Journal of Psychological Trauma*, 6(2–3), 35–63. doi: 10.1300/J513v06n02_04

Moskowitz, A. (2008). Association and dissociation in the historical concept of schizophrenia. In A. Moskowitz, I. Schäfer, & M.J. Dorahy, *Psychosis, trauma and dissociation: Emerging perspectives on severe psychopathology.* London: Wiley.

Moskowitz, A., & Heim, G. (2011). Eugen Bleuler's dementia praecox or the group of schizophrenias (1911): A centenary appreciation and reconsideration. *Schizophrenia Bulletin, 37*(3), 471–479.

Moskowitz, A., Heim, G., Saillot, I., & Beavan, V. (2019). Pierre Janet on hallucinations, paranoia, and schizophrenia. In G. Craparo, F. Ortu, O. van der Hart, (eds.), *Rediscovering Pierre Janet: Trauma, dissociation, and a new context for psychoanalysis.* New York: Routledge.

Myers, C.S. (1940). *Shell shock in France, 1914–1918.* Cambridge: Cambridge University Press.

Ratcliffe, M. (2017). *Real hallucinations: Psychiatric illness, intentionality, and the interpersonal world.* Cambridge: MIT.

Rhodes, J.E., Hackney, S.J., & Smith, J.A. (2019). Emptiness, engulfment, and life struggle: An interpretative phenomenological analysis of chronic depression. *Journal of Constructivist Psychology, 32*, 390–407.

Rowan, J. (2010). *Personification.* London: Routledge.

Sass, L.A., & Parnas, J. (2003). Schizophrenia, consciousness, and the self. *Schizophrenia Bulletin, 29*, 427–444.

Smith, J.A., & Rhodes, J.E. (2015). Being depleted and being shaken: An interpretative phenomenological analysis of the experiential features of a first episode of depression. *Psychology and Psychotherapy: Theory, Research, and Practice, 88*, 197–209.

Van der Hart, O., Niejenhuis, E., & Steele, K. (2006). *The haunted self: Structural dissociation and the treatment of chronic traumatisation.* New York: Norton.

Young, E., Klosko, J.S., & Weishaar, M.E. (2003). *Schema therapy: A practitioner's guide.* New York: Guilford Press.

7

COLLAPSE OF THE TAKEN-FOR-GRANTED WORLD

At many points in William's life he became convinced that terrorists and social services had set up an experiment of which he was the target. As part of this experiment he believed that he had been placed in a foster home as a spy. This account will, I believe, strike most readers as extraordinary if not impossible. It is interesting to note, however, that when well William himself found these ideas unbelievable and reported that the experience of being under their sway was terrible. The aim of this chapter is to analyse how such ideas and perceptions emerge and, in particular, to explore how abuse in childhood, or abuse to adults, contributes to psychosis and the formation of delusions and other psychotic meanings. It might have been expected, given the actual events of William's earlier years (chapter five), that in adult life he would be prone to straightforward ideas of being attacked or exploited by others; this would have been an obvious continuation of his experience and ideas into subsequent years. The question arises how his experiences and ideas became transformed in such an extraordinary manner.

DOI: 10.4324/9781003044956-7

Rhodes and Gipps (2008), drawing on theorists such as Jaspers (1963), argued that delusional experiences, when expressed as statements, imply ideas about the way the world works which normally would be regarded as impossible, even by the same person when in a non-delusional state. Furthermore, these delusional claims violate that which we take for granted. To illustrate this argument we can imagine what it might be like trying to persuade a sceptic who argues that since we have no sure knowledge at all, then what William says could be true or possible. William reported many strange and suspicious things, for example, an odd look given by a nurse or by several policemen on the same day. One could take each episode and give an everyday explanation. But once all the details of the specific experiences had been accounted for then a sceptic might still say that William's ideas seem logically possible and ask why they should not be true. One may struggle to answer this, but a possible response could be: in my experience most professionals can be trusted, within limits, and would be morally outraged by such an experiment, and therefore would not acquiesce to it. Of course, social services can make mistakes, and even break the law, but not on such a scale involving so many people for such a long time. Furthermore, while some people can be cruel, it is beyond belief that so many would participate in such abuse and not feel compelled to do something to stop it. To this argument the sceptic could still say: but it's possible, how do you know it did not happen? And for delusions involving extraordinary ideas such as time travel still say, but how do you know? After a lot of argument eventually we reach an end point, a limit of giving reasons, what in fact Wittgenstein (1969) called a 'bedrock' of everyday certainties beyond which one can go no further. To the sceptic we are reduced to making comments such as: well I just know most people are trustworthy within limits, that most people have compassion to some extent, and I just know that medical staff would not go along with a pointless and cruel plot even more so one from another country; furthermore, most people know this is the way the world is. If the sceptic persists, we still feel certain, yet may run out of words.

Wittgenstein explored forms of certainty as shown in our confidence that we exist, or that the world continues, or that people do not turn into trees. Moyal-Sharrock (2007), in developing Wittgenstein's arguments, suggested that such 'bedrock certainties' rest in the end on ways of living and acting in the world, and that it does not even make sense to ask us for the reasons why we maintain them. When we state a truth such as 'a person cannot walk through a solid wall', this is our attempt to put into words the non-reflective, living, certainties with which we act. The bedrock of our pre-verbal certainties is that which structures our behaviour in the presence of a wall or other solid surfaces: it is a set of behavioural and experiential dispositions. Since we have confidence facilitating dispositions, we are able to react to new situations in appropriate ways. Moyal-Sharrock suggests that trust and confidence also form part of a person's fundamental dispositions in the world. A key argument in this chapter will be that for those who become overwhelmed by persecutory delusions, and have histories of abuse, such trust and related certainties have been lost or were never developed.

The background and psychosis

In what follows I shall argue that delusions involve a suspension of that which Searle called 'the background' (1992) and draw on ideas given in Rhodes and Gipps (2008) and Fulford (1993). Searle originally presented this concept in his analysis of sentence meaning and intentionality, but then extended it as a general feature of meaning and action. The concept of the background overlaps with Wittgenstein's notion of bedrock certainties in that the latter form part of the background. The following is one specific argument for the background.

If we take any statement made in everyday English such as 'please make me a cup of coffee', then something is going very wrong if the person brings a cup full of coffee beans. To carry out the action as intended in context implies supplementary meanings; if we attempted to speculate what these might be, the following are possible: coffee here means not the original substance but a drink made by ground coffee beans brewed at a certain temperature following a specific method of production, or, it could mean a drink made with 'instant' coffee. What Searle observes, however, is that such ways of specifying the meaning never seem enough: each extra phrase adds new and open ways of interpreting the sentence, for example, what temperature exactly, how much water, within what timeframe should the drink be brought, etc. The process of explanation and justification seems without end; given this indeterminacy, Searle argues that eventually these meanings must rest on a background of ways of acting, taken for granted within a specific context and culture. In discussing meaning Searle notes how any specific beliefs about, for example, making coffee will tend to interconnect with many other beliefs; taken together, he calls these interconnected beliefs the network beyond which are the dispositions and abilities of the background.

Our background dispositions allow us to function in the world; as we approach a situation that may at first seem new, say, a first visit to a professional theatre, even without being given explicit rules we would know to listen, pay attention, to open any doors in order to walk through them, and that the performance onstage does not involve real blood and knives. Of course there are new things to learn such as whether to clap, when and to what degree; yet a vast number of behaviours, taken for granted and transferred from everyday life, are employed without thought. In psychology there has been a tendency to assume that all details of how people behave can be illuminated by cognitions and rules that we can specify; Searle and other philosophers have reversed this in suggesting that what is foundational is our skillful and meaningful action or behaviour in the world, and that our ability to generate cognitions, rests on this foundation of actions and dispositions.

Common sense as shared perspective

Blankenburg (2001) argued that in individuals with schizophrenia there is a loss of basic 'common sense'. Common sense here is not meant to be just sensible advice, for example, 'don't get into debt', but rather an ability to cope in the everyday practical and social world. It is a sense of what the appropriate thing might be to do as we try to manage and interact with others. He quotes participants who articulated how they felt that they had lost this ability. One said: 'what is it that I'm missing? ... I have lost a hold in regard to the simplest everyday things. It seems that I lack a natural understanding for what is matter of course and obvious to others'. This participant went on to give examples such as how to behave on the ward and how to just be with others.

Blankenburg argues, at least during severe episodes of psychosis, that individuals feel they have lost some kind of sense of how to be and how to do things in the everyday world. Stanghellini (2004) has also developed the argument that schizophrenia involves the disappearance of common sense ability. Blankenburg describes how several writers have attempted to articulate what this common sense might be and draws on Kant who argued for a connection between mental illness and common sense. Blankenburg selects two key quotes from Kant (the translations I use here are taken from Scholten, 2016): 'the only universal characteristic of madness is the loss of common sense (sensus communis) and its replacement with logical private sense (sensus privatus).' Of particular importance, however, is how Kant defines commonsense: 'by sensus communis should be understood the idea of a communal sense, i.e., a faculty for judging that in its reflection takes account (a priori) of everyone else's way of representing in thought in order as it were to hold its judgement up to human reason as a whole and thereby avoid illusion.' Scholten goes on to argue that for Kant mental illness involved the 'loss of a shared world'.

The notion of the background and the notion of common sense ability clearly overlap. Common sense or shared sense might be defined as those abilities needed for the everyday collective world and ones facilitated by background capacities and dispositions. Furthermore, articulating the fact that this sense takes into consideration the views of others, we might say that common sense is supported by diverse persons employing a shared background. However unique and idiosyncratic a person's particular background capacities are, they must involve a sensitivity to shared situations and social practices; given the commonality of situations, one might predict that a considerable part, if not the majority, of a person's background is shared to some extent with others, and that this sharing of distributed backgrounds within a specific culture is key to social life and a sense of 'what is the case'.

Fuchs (2020) in recent papers has outlined an intersubjective and enactivist conception of delusions. He argues that everyday perception of the social world involves action and exploration of that world, and requires that the perspective of others is taken into account. Fuchs observes that as a person becomes psychotic he or she loses the very capacity to share a perspective, and to construct meaning in participating with others. Eventually this ends in what he calls 'subjectivisation': the person is at the centre of things, chance events and overheard comments are about that person. As the person moves into deeper psychosis, then the capacity to differentiate 'it is as if I am being followed' from ' I am ...' is lost and connection to common sense and background is altered.

Fuchs argues that his work is focused on perception and inter-subjectivity, noting that the changes described by Sass and Parnas (2003), such as self awareness and agency, are an alternative though overlapping route and may lead to similar end points, in particular, a collapse of the ability to differentiate 'as if' and the loss of background. It may be that the routes described in this chapter, that is, of child and adult abuse, are additional ones and may or may not overlap.

Psychosis and social experience

While the background dispositions of a person are an interconnected system, subsets of dispositions may concern different areas of living and have degrees of depth (Searle, 1992). To cope and manage in the world we need to relate to diverse entities and features which include: other people; the world of everyday human made objects such as chairs, computers, cars; physical and biological properties as given in our everyday experience, for example, that floors are hard, that animals move and eat food. While delusions can include a very wide range of themes, such as invented technologies and extraordinary changes in biology or physical properties, most have a social and relational focus (Rhodes, Jakes & Robinson, 2005; Rhodes & Jakes, 2010) and may be said to relate to the social aspects of background capacity.

In normal social interaction we see others, we think about them, we react and have a complex range of changing feelings about what is going on. When a person is paranoid all these processes and reactions are also taking place but are now imbued with the conceptions and feelings of persecution and, for example, concern with what plot may be taking place. A person may see someone who gives a 'strange look'; for the person with paranoia this is yet another example of the actions of those who have been in pursuit over several months and relates to an ultimate conspiracy. The person feels strange, watched, judged, particularly in delusion-relevant situations (e.g., this might be a policeman on the street or one of many difficult neighbours). The action of the other is suspicious. There are often purported coincidences between the behaviours of diverse persons; one client mentioned the extraordinary number of road works by a specific company on his routes. The sufferer does not feel safe and feels no trust or confidence in what others are doing.

In the context of receiving therapy participants were asked what they had witnessed or felt that week which made them continue to maintain their beliefs (Rhodes & Jakes, 2004); most listed specific observations such as given above and then explained how these events were obviously part of the ongoing plot. By far the most common support for claims involved reporting what others were observed to be doing in specific situations. There were of course other sources; one being the episodic hearing of voices, but this too often involves a relationship with the hallucinated entity. Paranoia is fundamentally social and involves suspicion and the absence of trust.

The nature of trust

Moyal-Sharrock suggests that trust can be seen as a form of certainty. The importance of trust for psychosis has been explored by Earnshaw (2011), Ratcliffe, Ruddell, and Smith (2014), and Ratcliffe (2017). Trust is something we do and feel and not usually thought about; as Moyal-Sharrock points out, we may only come to realise that we did trust someone when trust is lost. It is not something we usually try to express as rules, but rather we have a sense of how, and to what extent, we can trust others. Sometimes we do make a specific statement such as 'yes, I trust this person', but to attempt to specify a set of 'rules' for how and to what degree we can trust different persons with different things is extremely difficult, if possible at all. For example, could we trust a stranger with a small or large sum of money? Can we trust a friend who we have known only a few months, and if not, how many months or years are needed? When does the change occur? I believe that such 'rules' are mere speculation, unsuccessful approximations that attempt to capture our complex evolving behavior. Yet, although we cannot articulate a set of clear guidelines for 'how and when to trust', our actions do seem to instantiate a coherent pattern, and most people just know what to do. For topics such as trust we have a 'feel', a sense of what is appropriate in specific situations. Trust overlaps with the concept of common sense as noted earlier. The overlap underlines how trust is not an idiosyncratic list of 'dos and don'ts' but involves a practice in a social context with a shared perspective. Baier (1986) and Moyal-Sharrock both suggest that trust is something seen in the behavior of infants with their parents. Within a bond of trust, learning about the world and what others are like is facilitated. If a child is abused, then this will have a severe impact on the development of trust and also learning. I return to the relevance of trust later sections.

The delusions of William, that he had been a spy, an 'experiment', a target over decades, imply claims that violate our collective background. Looking at the various implications of his delusions, one major feature was of trust. The more he became unwell, the less trust he had in others. As argued above, trust is not just a set of rules or ideas he could articulate. Trust is a tendency to act in certain trusting ways. In everyday life our world feels 'trustworthy', at least within limits and in certain contexts: this was not the case for William when unwell. In a state of emotional distress, his fear-driven imagination threw out ever more unpleasant and extreme ideas and during that time his background dispositions did not allow him to reject these ideas, to ground him back in the everyday world.

Other aspects of the background

Rhodes and Gipps (2008) outlined several features of experience relating to background functioning, which included differentiation of the real and unreal, the self and non-self, the capacity to differentiate literal from metaphorical statements. Fuchs, as described, argues that in the onset of psychosis the person loses the sense of 'as if'; such alterations indicate a change in the functioning of the background. The relevance of distinguishing literal from non-literal during psychosis was also discussed in chapter five.

In this chapter I have focused in particular on the concept of background dispositions and Wittgenstein's bedrock certainties. Some theorists, however, have used other conceptions: Dreyfus (1995), drawing on Heidegger, articulated how a person has an 'understanding of being' and that the latter is not an explicit cognitive activity but something realised in the way the person lives. Stanghellini (2004) also employs ideas from Heidegger in his way of approaching psychosis and common sense.

What might lead the background to change during psychosis?

In Rhodes and Gipps (2008), we speculated on how the background might change in psychosis and considered the possible contribution of a biological route. Friston and Frith (1995) presented a model describing how in order for normal functioning of the brain to work subtle and complex interconnections of many areas are required; psychosis is seen as a product of the breakdown or alteration in these functional interconnections. We speculated that such neurological patterns might realise or instantiate on a neurological level the global complexity of background functioning; likewise, a suspension of background in psychosis might be realised on the neurological level by a disturbance of interconnected coherence.

We also considered how abuse and early experiences might be a possible route to background alterations, and how social and emotional conditions of childhood, in particular situations which could induce a disturbance of trust, may in turn have an influence in later years on the formation of delusions. In one case illustration we noted how a man with paranoia had experienced as a child daily bombardment of intrusive questions by his mother concerning his behaviour and that of others; a sort of daily interrogation in which his mother displayed deep mistrust. In another case a man had grown up with a father who had claimed he was a pope. In the first case trust in others was undermined and in the second case there appeared to be the creation of a background at odds with the surrounding society and one leading to a readiness to accept extraordinary claims. Both cases involved emotional abuse and mistreatment. In the rest of this chapter I will further develop how trauma might influence the onset of psychosis by its impact upon those features described above, that is, of the background, trust, of common sense certainties, and shared perspectives.

Exploring the effects of abuse and their relation to the background

In following four sections I shall argue that the evidence presented illustrates the effects of abuse and ones which indicate that the background has been changed. I will summarise how trust was mentioned as a theme by most participants in earlier chapters and then look at confusion, followed by credulity and the acceptance of extraordinary ideas. Finally I will look at evidence that indicates how a person's capacity to understand social reality had been disturbed in early years.

Loss of trust

Concerning trust it is striking that this was a clearly articulated theme across all three groups of participants, that is, the physically abused, the sexually abused, and refugees. Here I will select just a few representative examples. Of those with histories of physical abuse Chris stated 'I don't trust people' while Greg said 'trust was lost'. Of those with histories of sexual abuse Tony stated 'I can't trust anybody' while Sue said 'I don't feel the trust'. Examples from those who were refugees included Togar saying 'I don't have trust' and Sando who stated that it was 'very hard... to trust'. Some of the refugees described how this state of lacking trust was new and developed after their traumas.

Without trust and a shared perspective, the extraordinary is possible.

Observing the presence of psychosis in those who have undergone extreme trauma such as torture, Ratcliffe, Ruddell, and Smith (2014) argue that the destruction of trust takes away a person's capacity for a shared perspective, the latter being that which facilitates a sense of what is the case or otherwise. They describe how our beliefs are embedded in a dependable and predictable public world; other people have a 'regulatory role' and our relationship with others influences our experiences, thoughts, and future projects. Our beliefs are shaped by interactions with others, and when this is altered the very way beliefs are formed or maintained will change. Changes in trust and our relations may even influence a sense of what is real and the boundaries between self and others, which in turn opens the person to the possibility of hallucinations and delusions. They also comment on how a change in trust will involve an alteration in the predictability of everyday life and may have relevance in understanding 'aberrant salience' as conceptualised by Kapur (2003), that is, how, for those with psychosis, mundane things can suddenly seem very important and demand attention. In Ratcliffe (2017) the above arguments are expanded, including the relevance of habitual certainties and the background.

Confusion and not knowing

Several comments made by the participants suggested alterations in thinking and states of mind where the person could not be sure of knowing what was happening, usually concerning others. What is noticed by the person seems disconnected and remains just appearances, ungrounded, and one does not know what is really happening.

In general, the comments focused on social events. Zoe stated, concerning her relationship with a boyfriend, 'I get confused' and when talking about the motivations of others added 'you don't know whether it's reality or not sometimes'. Jackie described the time in her life when she heard that her daughter had been raped at which point she 'lost reality and everything…I was thinking not, you know, not real at all' and later added 'it was all like a dream'. Merza said that, following his breakdown, his 'whole way of thinking is different', and 'you don't know what's inside anyone's head'; here there is a combination of lack of trust and lack of knowing. Toni gave the sweeping statement: 'nobody knows what goes on in the mind'.

Several comments by the refugee group also indicated not knowing: Belvie said that it was '…difficult for me… the difference between a dream and reality'. Lionel described a time when he thought he was being followed in the UK 'when it was like a dream'. Amine was not sure if a black cat he had seen was 'real' or not. He also reported seeing a disturbing portrait in the hospital which he had experienced as if animated: a man appeared to begin to come out of it. However, in describing this he seemed puzzled and unsure.

The comments above suggest that the participants were unsure of what was happening around them; furthermore, they sometimes experienced themselves as being in altered states which seemed disconnected or dreamlike. Van der Hart, Niejenhuis, and Steele (2006) developing ideas from Janet argued that trauma fundamentally involves the loss of the capacity for 'realisation' and that normal consciousness and interaction not only require the ability to bring together and synthesise ideas but that the person must be able to grasp such fundamental realities as being in the here and now (termed 'presentification') and to know what is self and not self (termed 'personalisation'). The capacity for realisation is altered due to the effects of trauma. Other examples of non-realisation given by van der Hart include not knowing that it was oneself who did an action or believing that a past action is occurring in the present.

It is noteworthy that the same sorts of fundamental confusions and disorientations are found in both psychosis and PTSD and may involve similar changes. From a background theory perspective the sorts of experiences generated by the processes of realisation such as knowing something is present and real are not ones we arrive at by conscious thought. Rather, these are automatic processes that we take for granted and which produce our experience. Given 'realisation' involves background capacity, so its loss is another example of how trauma alters a person's background and might contribute to the process of becoming psychotic. The contribution of non-realisation involves the separation or suspension of functions and this fits the model of disconnection, outlined by Bleuler (1950), involving the disconnection of psychological and neuro-cognitive functions and processes.

Credulity and unanchored thinking

While the above comments indicate not knowing, the following almost suggests the opposite in that the person was too ready to believe ideas or experiences of persecution and other sorts of delusion. Several comments describe a sort of concatenation of paranoid meanings and experiencing these as persuasive. The ideas seem somehow unanchored, too certain, revelatory, and full of meaning. William stated how 'it all makes sense' when he is becoming unwell, and Chris reported that he came to 'conclusions' and that he has 'associative thinking'. Lesley, with physical abuse, stated about others 'everything they say I'll twist up' and that she 'becomes so fixated on everything'. Clare stated concerning difficult situations 'every thought...you buy into it' and that she regarded herself as 'gullible'.

Two general points concerning unanchored thinking; first, the moments of idea generation and distress occurred in both extreme psychotic episodes, but also sometimes in everyday social reactions of the person. Second, how the person got into such states of distress may involve different routes such as anxiety, overwhelming emotions, hyper-arousal, and driven states perhaps involving salience; these were discussed in earlier chapters.

The participants' statements suggest that not only are extreme ideas generated but that these are experienced as immediately sure and display a sort of credulity. Whether for one or many diverse details noticed by the person, in this way of thinking, the wider context is disengaged both in terms of relevant accessible ideas, but also a felt sense of what is possible and real, indicating a disconnection of background. As noted earlier, without background and trust, the mundane will already seem different and strange prompting attempts to explain; but if a person is in a very disturbed emotional state, particularly concerning long-standing areas of distress, then the person may be too ready to believe any generated idea or image. It is precisely the background which should give the person a sense of the reality or unreality of distorted and extreme imagination.

The evidence in chapter two pointed to the importance of episodic transformations of accelerating anxiety, disturbance, and a complete change in mental state or consciousness. Whether feelings of anxiety emerge from ordinary concerns or paranoid ideas and experience, the anxiety itself will further narrow attention and focus the individual on possible threats and worst-case scenarios (Eysenck et al., 2007). The feelings of dread combined with unanchored ideas may then create a vicious cycle producing a sort of psychotic panic. The person ends up being increasingly certain about the extraordinary, the dreamlike if not nightmarish world of imagined persecution, but uncertain and adrift concerning mundane everyday interactions and cut off from any reassurance or help others could provide.

Trauma and modes of intentionality

Some of the evidence above indicates a shift in the person's capacity to maintain a grasp on imagination, conjecture, and in contrast, the perception of what is real. One argument exploring trauma and psychosis developed by Ratcliffe (2017) concerns intentionality and how it functions. He stated that different sorts of intentional states, such as perceiving or imagining, have distinctive patterns of anticipation and fulfillment that unfold over time, that is to say, we anticipate certain things and these are satisfied or not in appropriate ways. If we turn away for a second from seeing a table, we expect that it will still be there when we look again and that other people have continued to see it. In contrast, if we imagine a table, then it is not surprising if the table turns from wood to gold, whatever our imagination carries out, but we would not expect others to be able to see what we are imaging.

Certainty and confidence are foundational in how we actually perceive things and how we are able to differentiate that which is perceived in contrast to imagined or remembered. But if a person is emotionally disturbed in a situation and feels uncertain, then the boundaries between perceiving and imagining may become unstable and permeable. Ratcliffe also links these changes with possible alterations in the background and everyday habitual certainties, as argued earlier in this chapter, and with a breakdown in a person's capacity to share perspectives.

Putting the ideas of this section and the last one together suggests that those with psychosis have lost their normal certainties for many everyday topics, and when something induces disturbance or terror, or if the person for whatever reason is already in a highly aroused and driven state, then the imagined or just supposed appears as pressing, sure, full of meaning. Furthermore, the latter are increased by the force of immediate experiences and undergone without the breaking force of former certainties concerning both what has been imagined (how a fictional entity might behave) and on a person's capacity to automatically know and be sure they are or are not engaging in acts of imagination. The person comes to inhabit an imagination transformed world with delusional certainties based on immediate disturbing experience.

Abuse of the capacity to know and learn

For some forms of abuse, particularly sexual abuse, there was often a direct threat used to prevent the sufferer telling anyone about what was going on. There were also situations when a child might have known something was taking place in their family, but was threatened and told to remain silent, and sometimes even the child's capacity to know was denied. In yet other families, the assault on knowing was not stated bluntly but the child experienced severe contrasts between what was seen and what was said in the family. In short, the interviews suggested in diverse ways that a person's ability to know was compromised. Of course in the context of abuse it is extremely likely that the harm inflicted upon the ability to know and trust, or the creation of mistrust, was a process that took place over many years.

Examples from those with physical abuse

Peter:

> Something didn't't ring true you know, it was, all this talk of love and God and all this stuff, umm, and we weren't't seeing any of it. Now, I would see my brother and sister being swung round and round the bedroom by their hair you know?

Lesley:

And then another time I called the police because he was on top on her by the corner of this room and pushing her head against this corner and shaking her, pulling her hair, but I jumped on his back, scratched him, pulled his hair and he, he just wouldn't't let go of her. So I called the police and the police came, he chucked pasta everywhere and umm, then he said, then my mum said "oh nothing's happening, it was just a falling out, and I started the argument" and then my dad went "yeah, she mad, that girl's mad" and umm.

Interviewer:

Was this when you were quite young?

Lesley:

Yeah, I was very young about 7 or 8. My mum and dad spilt up when I was 12.

William:

I think the first time (that is when he was beaten) I thought I'd done something wrong or you know what, I was confused really… I thought I must have done something wrong but I couldn't see in myself what I'd done wrong.

Later he added:

I was in a situation where I was regretful about everything had happened, not really accepting that I'd been at fault, yet agreeing that I might have been at fault.

Examples from sexual abuse

Sue stated about the abuse:

I felt a bit alienated, I felt. I didn't know what was going on. I was blaming myself rather than the person who was doing it to me.

When Clare told her mother about the sexual abuse, she took Clare to confront her father and the following took place:

And so I told him exactly the way it was. And umm, he jumped out of bed. Grabbed his belt from his jeans at the bottom of the bed and started swinging this belt all over me. Just literally bang, bang, bang, bang all over me. I don't know how many times. Twenty, thirty times maybe. And umm, I'm trying to get out of the room. I keep trying to get to the door to get out. Frightened, really frightened, and it hurts obviously. I'm trying to get out the door, but my mum she keeps grabbing hold of me and pushing me back towards him. She's not protecting me at all and, umm, he didn't say a word. He didn't say 'you're lying' and he didn't say 'this isn't true' he didn't say anything. He just, as I say, hit me with this belt over and over again. And then my mum said to me 'right, now go to your room'. And umm, so I went into my room, and I sat there and I cried and cried and cried. And I think from that moment on I just decided even if it happens again I'll never tell anybody. And so I, and so then the next day they bought me this gift, umm, umm, a knitting needle set. And they said, this is because you haven't wet your bed.

What does such an episode do to a person? What version of reality is being created here? Such events, besides being deeply upsetting and traumatic, strike at the very core of a person's grasp of what is taking place and ability to share the truth. The events isolate the person: to tell the truth is to risk violent and potentially life-threatening attack.

For some there was a clear threat that no one must be told. Lesley stated, 'I had to keep it a secret'. Irene was told she would be beaten, and Sue that if she said anything the family would break up. These are extraordinary threats for a young person. The very means by which they could make sense of things, and of sharing their agony, were denied to them.

These biographical incidents are horrific, and remind us of the extremity of what children go through. For those who have grown up with secure childhoods, such episodes are almost beyond imagination. Children not only form specific memories at such times but learn something about the nature of the world and what other humans are like. The conclusion that others can be dangerous and cannot be trusted may well be deeply fused into the person's fundamental expectations about the world.

Epistemic trust and the ability to learn

The role of trust in the learning of children has been explored by Koenig and Harris (2007) and Sperber et al. (2010), who developed the concept of epistemic trust, that is, the capacity of a person to differentiate what information is trustworthy and worthwhile in a situation of being exposed to multiple and sometimes conflicting information. Sperber and colleagues describe how a child, for efficient learning, needs to assume and trust that the knowledge being taught is shared and important. In approaching learning, children will be concerned with not only content but the source of that content. Efficient learning requires that we trust the source of that learning and what is being taught is shared by the community.

Fonagy, Luyten, and Allison (2015) note how learning is fostered in the context of attachment between child and adult and this is where mentalisation, the capacity to understand oneself and others, is simultaneously being developed. However, they also underline the importance of communication and epistemic trust. They argue that this capacity has been harmed in children who have received mistreatment and that this contributes to the development of borderline personality disorder. Such adults remain trapped in that they cannot trust information that suggests newly encountered environments or persons might be benign or that prior extreme negative expectations no longer hold.

A potential link between abuse, epistemic mistrust, and psychosis has been outlined by Ratcliffe (2017). It seems likely that the same sort of processes and factors given above also apply in the development of children who have been abused and then go on to develop psychosis; that is, adults abused as children will have profound epistemic mistrust, will continue to be trapped in the expectation of mistreatment, and will find it very difficult to learn in a new environment—such as a therapeutic relationship—that others can be trusted and that there are new things to learn. The idea that abused children may have difficulties with some types of learning is consistent with other research (Toth et al., 2011) demonstrating that young children who have suffered abuse had difficulties with types of reasoning involved in story comprehension and had a tendency to misinterpret the behaviour of others as threatening.

The effects of abuse on epistemic trust will be multiple and take place over many years; in the evidence given above, however, we see particularly extreme examples of a direct attack on the capacity to know. These reports are however just the most conspicuous explicit memories of a long-term process, most of which could not be put into words.

Overview of the findings

Putting the four strands of evidence together, we might say that the participants as adults lived in a world where they could not trust others, were often confused about what was happening, and yet sometimes experienced persuasive imagination concerning threat. Furthermore, they had had experiences as children which had curtailed or even destroyed the capacity of being open to new information, such that in adult years the person became unable to find a way out of confusion and mistrust. If trauma has an influence on psychosis by affecting a person's background capacities, then how might this develop over time for children as opposed to adults? I will first explore the experience of those who have suffered trauma as adults, and then the experience of adults traumatised as children.

Development of psychosis in those abused as adults

Adults who have been subject to extreme political violence, or other kinds of abuse such as domestic abuse, often report, as described earlier, a severe collapse in trust and a transformation of expectations concerning what the world and other people are like. What was taken for granted, for example, that the world is safe, that others can be trusted, and that help would be given if in distress, all these are violated. The change the person undergoes is not just about developing different explicit ideas concerning safety; rather, they have experienced a severe alteration of their background dispositional capacities to trust and have faith in the world. As argued in this chapter, without trust a person can begin to find credible new extreme ideas about what others are doing.

Abuse strikes at the very core of a person's capacity to trust and violates a person's capacity to develop a shared perspective with others. How could one even begin to investigate what is going on if the other cannot be trusted, that is, if no one can be trusted to share one's thought with. For the abused there is no 'we' and therefore there cannot be a base from which one could even begin to feel a sense of what was possible and not possible, reasonable or not reasonable. Further, it is not just a question of actually talking to others; the person will also not be able to generate a sense of a trustworthy 'other' in imagination, explicitly or implicitly, to engage in a sort of internal dialogue using the perspective of another (this point was discussed by Blankenburg).

Broken self and the grasp of the real

In the data for refugees a significant theme was that of the 'broken self'. The participants were very clear in saying that they were no longer, in some profound way, the same person. This I believe is quite similar to the experience of an altered self as found in long-term depression (Rhodes, Hackney & Smith, 2019) as presented in chapter six. It was also argued in chapter six that we can conceptualise the person as not in fact being constituted by just one personality state but rather that a person may have a repertoire of possible selves or personality states. Given the person may have such a repertoire then it might well be that these different states have differential access to the global background of the person, and in particular, some states will be substantially disengaged from normal everyday background; in non-psychotic depression it is not rare to come across barely credible claims such as that one will soon be 'living on the street' in spite of being financially secure and having a supportive family.

I would suggest that a terrified self or destabilising rage might well be the states of self most disconnected from background. For the majority of traumatised individuals, however, the coping self will have a just about good enough access to the background, though not necessarily a full access as the person had before trauma. The more distressed parts of the self, however, will tend to have only partial access or fluctuating access according to how distressing any particular situation might be. The person in the state of threat is highly focused on the specific task of self protection or escape: there is no room at that point for any flexible consideration of multiple interpretations. The person will attend narrowly and selectively to threat (Eysenck et al., 2007), at the expense of a perspective involving the viewpoints of others.

In sum, torture and other forms of adult abuse have diverse effects, including terror, rage, hopelessness, and often depression; trauma also leads to the destruction of the person's capacity to trust. The extreme negative emotional states of terror and anger will tend to be cut off from the person's former background, how the person is grounded in the everyday shared world. Experiencing fluctuating states of distress, loss of one's former lived identity, loss of context, a sense of non-realisation, loss of others, and all these being experienced without connection to the former background, the person may increasingly believe their worst fears and the products of imagination concerning danger from others, even to the point of psychotic persecutory delusion. Intermingled with the effects of dread, mistrust, and loss, traumatised individuals also frequently experience varying depths of depression, which adds further disturbance and undermines the functioning and just about coping self.

Development of psychosis in those abused as children

How might child abuse lead to psychosis? In particular, if the abuse suffered is causal, then why is it that often the effects of abuse seem to lie dormant for years before the emergence of psychosis? To answer this I think we need first to draw on ideas concerning abuse and child development presented by trauma theorists such as Van der Hart, Niejenhuis, and Steele (2006) and Fisher (2017). It is suggested that those who have been abused during childhood develop a way of being with others, such that the person will have severe vulnerabilities or limitations but can at least cope with the world in conventional situations; however, given the extremity of mistreatment there will also develop parts of the self that experience terror or shame. Fisher (2017) argues that such a person may well manage during years of early adulthood but in situations of extreme distress, fear, or depression, the everyday coping self will be suspended and the person will come to be dominated by sub-parts of personality which incorporate mistrust, dread, and anticipate attack. To this developmental picture I wish to add that the self in terror or rage will not be able to access the wider foundation of personal capacities or world orientated know-how, will not be able to trust, nor will the capacity to see things from the other's perspective be developed: that is, the very conditions likely to facilitate the onset of psychosis.

Carson McCullars (1961) writes: 'But the hearts of small children are delicate organs.' The abused child is deeply wounded and 'learns' many things: that others cannot be trusted, that those who 'care' might deceive, might attack, can be dangerous, that the world can be full of pain and dread and no one will help. The child learns mistrust at the deepest level;

some aspects might be expressible in words, but this mistrust will be, above all, a disposition to act and react. The child also develops the capacity to dissociate in order to bear the pain, to somehow survive the 'madness' of what is being inflicted upon them. As the biographic episodes given above indicate, the actual world for these children was often incomprehensible, dangerous, and dominated by the erratic and frightening actions of adults. They were forced to experience that what they 'knew' or 'saw' as real to be not real, since that was what the adults told them. Furthermore, as children tend to blame themselves, they came to believe that they must be at fault or defective in their ways of seeing the world. To blame oneself in these contexts, however, is already a distortion of reality and truth. Furthermore, without the capacity for epistemic trust, the young person and adult may become blocked from new learning, therefore allowing the perpetuation of an assumed world of danger.

In parallel with abuse, however, children can also be immersed in another world of normal predictable actions and caring adults; these diverse 'worlds' can exist simultaneously. Abuse is often episodic. There are is, of course, a multitude of possible developmental pathways; some children are treated well for years, but then exposed to sexual abuse or violence in teenage years from step-parents or neighbours. Other children are, most of the time, in relatively safe and predictable environments, but there are sometimes sudden attacks from an out of control raging parent. In other cases there might well be a caring father or mother but the other parent has periodic storms of rage and attack. A child learns to adapt to these complex contradictory worlds and may have to develop sub-personalities to fit within the challenging environment. Children on the whole seem to develop some capacity to cope in times of relative peace, such as at school where they may find relative safety. It is this just about coping self which gets the child through school and sometimes allows the person to start work. But in depression, or accumulated states of fear, this coping self disintegrates and reveals not just a vulnerable self, but one full of terror, suspicion, and dread. Others are seen as threatening, and almost any type of imagined strange behavior by others is taken to be feasible; it then seems persuasive that there is a gang plotting ones destruction and members of the gang are disguised as policemen on the street. Some children, however, who are immersed in extreme environments, with almost no positive experiences, do not manage to develop a coping self, or at best form a fragile minimal version, and can display forms of suffering from a young age, including psychotic features.

Many of those who are abused not only develop fearful terrified parts of self but also have extreme ideas or expectations about others. They have seen and felt the terrible presence of the attacking other. As the adult survivor becomes anxious or depressed, and the terrified child part begins to predominate, then connected to this will be implicit and explicit memories of the attacking other. It is these past and transformed memories which imbue with meaning the person's perception of the attacking 'gang', the terrible organisation engaged in cruel plots, others who express contempt, or the threats expressed in persecutory voices and attacking entities.

To recap, as a person becomes psychotic, the coping self, fragile or otherwise, is disconnected from its background, and in addition, for those with child abuse, a terror state of self comes to predominate, one with not only memories of abuse but also a background developed in the abusive environment, that is, one that carries with it dispositions attuned to the particular and disturbing 'world' as experienced by the child. An adult functioning with such a background is open to the acceptance of un-realistic and terrible possibilities.

The impacts of adult trauma and child abuse, though having distinct features as described above, have at their core the same crucial steps, that is, abuse leads to the destruction of trust and the creation of dread; this constitutes a change in the person's global background, that is, the set of capacities which normally ground the person in the everyday shared world. Without the capacity to sense, in an immediate way, the improb-ability of extreme ideas, delusions, and other psychotic content can be both generated and believed. Concerning hallucinations, the very ex-pectations of attack from the other, formed during abuse and held by a vulnerable part of self, leads to the seeing or hearing of a recreated at-tacking entity.

Summary

Throughout this book I have argued that trauma has a wide range of ef-fects. Some of these are conspicuous, such as changes in emotions, cog-nitions and behaviours, while other effects require more analysis to specify their relevance. These consequences may include the suspension of every day habitual certainties, loss of trust, fragmentation of the self, confusion and not knowing, loss of the capacity for realisation, credulity and un-anchored ideas, lack of epistemic trust, and for some individuals, periodic depression involving the suspension or destruction of coping lived iden-tity. I have argued that several of the effects of trauma point to an alteration in the person's background capacities and dispositions, including those that facilitate everyday taken for granted ways of interacting and per-ceiving: in fact, how we exist in the world. To the extent that trauma begins to deeply alter background capacities that ground the person in the shared world, the person will be prone to states of psychosis. Children who have been traumatised may develop compartmentalised states of self such as being in extreme terror, and which can lay dormant until un-leashed by the challenges and stresses of adult life. In the next two chapters, I will turn to the possibility of psychological therapy for helping those who have experienced such states.

References

Baier, A. (1986). Trust and antitrust. *Ethics, 96,* 231–260.

Blankenburg, W. (2001). First steps toward a psychopathology of "common sense." (1969) (Transl. A. Mishara). *Philosophy, Psychiatry, and Psychology, 8,* 303–315.

Bleuler, E. (1950). *Dementia praecox or the group of schizophrenias.* New York: International Universities Press.

Dreyfus, H.L. (1995). *Being-in-the-world: a commentary on Heidegger's being and time. Division 1.* Cambridge: MIT Press.

Earnshaw, O. (2011). Recovering the voice of insanity: A phenomenology of delusions. Ph.D. thesis, Durham, University. Available at Durham E-Theses online: http://etheses.dur.ac.uk/3225/.

Eysenck, M.W., Derakshan, N., Santos, R., & Calvo, M.G. (2007). Anxiety and cognitive performance: Attentional control theory. *Emotion, 7*(2), 336–353.

Fisher, J. (2017). *Healing the fragmented selves of trauma survivors.* New York: Routledge.

Fonagy, P., Luyten, P., & Allison, E. (2015). Epistemic petrification and the restoration of epistemic trust: A new conceptualization of borderline personality disorder and its psychosocial treatment. *Journal of Personality Disorders, 29*(5), 575–609.

Friston, K.J., & Frith, C.D. (1995). Schizophrenia - a disconnection syndrome. *Clinical Neuroscience, 3*, 89–97.

Fuchs, T. (2020). Delusion, reality, and intersubjectivity: A Phenomenological and enactive analysis. *Philosophy, Psychiatry, & Psychology, 27*(1), 61–79.

Fulford, K.W.M. (1993). Mental illness and the mind-brain problem: Delusion, belief and Searle's theory of intentionality. *Theoretical Medicine, 14*, 181–194.

Gross, C.S. (2004). Struggling with imaginaries of trauma and trust: The refugee experience in Switzerland. *Cultural Medicine and Psychiatry, 28*, 151–167.

Jaspers, K. (1963, originally published in 1913) *General Psychopathology* (Transl. J. Hoenig and M. Hamilton). Manchester: Manchester University Press.

Kapur. S. (2003). Psychosis as a state of aberrant salience: A framework linking biology, phenomenology, and pharmacology in schizophrenia. *American Journal of Psychiatry, 160*, 13–23.

Koenig, M.A., &. Harris, P.L. (2007). The Basis of epistemic trust: Reliable testimony or reliable sources? *Episteme: A Journal of Social Epistemology, 4*(3), 264–284.

McCullars, C. (1961). *The Ballad of the Sad Café*. London: Penguin.

Moyal-Sharrock, D. (2007). *Understanding Wittgenstein's on certainty*. Basingstoke: Palgrave Macmillan.

Ratcliffe, M. (2015). *Experiences of depression*. Oxford: OUP.

Ratcliffe, M. (2017). *Real hallucinations: psychiatric illness, intentionality, and the interpersonal world*. Cambridge: MIT Press.

Ratcliffe, M., Ruddell, M., & Smith, B. (2014). What is a "sense of foreshortened future?" A phenomenological study of trauma, trust, and time. *Frontiers in Psychology, 5*, 1–11.

Rhodes, J.E., Hackney, S.J., & Smith, J.A. (2019). Emptiness, engulfment, and life struggle: An interpretative phenomenological analysis of chronic depression. *Journal of Constructivist Psychology, 32*(4), 390–407.

Rhodes, J., & Gipps, R. (2008). Delusions, certainty, and the background. *Philosophy, Psychiatry, and Psychology, 15*(4), 295–310.

Rhodes, J.E., & Jakes, S.C. (2004). Evidence given for delusions during cognitive behaviour therapy. *Clinical Psychology and Psychotherapy, 11*, 207–218.

Rhodes, J., Jakes, S., & Robinson, J. (2005). A qualitative analysis of delusional content. *Journal of Mental Health*, 14(4), 383–398.

Rhodes, J.E., & Jakes, S. (2010). Perspectives on the onset of delusions. *Clinical Psychology and Psychotherapy*, 17(2), 136–146.

Scholten, M. (2016). Schizophrenia and moral responsibility: A Kantian essay. *Philosophia*, 44, 205–225.

Sass, L.A., & Parnas, J. (2003). Schizophrenia, consciousness, and the self. *Schizophrenia Bulletin*, 29, 427–444.

Searle, J.R. (1992). *The rediscovery of the mind*. Cambridge: MIT Press.

Sperber, D., Clement, F., Heintz, C., Mascaro, O., Mercier, H., Origgi, G., & Wilson, D. (2010). Epistemic vigilance. *Mind & Language*, 25(4), 359–393.

Stanghellini, G. (2004). *Disembodied spirits and deanimated bodies: The psychopathology of common sense*. Oxford: OUP.

Toth, S. L., Pickreign Stronach, E., Rogosch, F. A., Caplan, R., & Cicchetti, D. (2011). Illogical thinking and thought disorder in maltreated children. *Journal of the American Academy of Child and Adolescent Psychiatry*, 50, 659–668.

Van der Hart, O., Niejenhuis, E., & Steele, K. (2006). *The haunted self: Structural dissociation and the treatment of chronic traumatisation*. New York: Norton.

Wittgenstein, L. (1969). *On certainty*. Oxford: Blackwell Publishers.

8

THERAPY FOR PSYCHOSIS AND TRAUMA

The aim of this and the next chapter is to consider whether therapeutic approaches that use a version of states of the self might be useful in the context of psychosis and trauma. Several therapies have now been developed for working with persons who have suffered both abuse and experience long-term interpersonal difficulties, and such therapies may well be a fruitful area to draw upon for working with psychosis.

Overview of findings and analysis

First I wish to summarise the key findings and concepts from the previous chapters. When we compare the meaning found in those with sexual and physical abuse it becomes apparent that the type of trauma not only influences every day meanings, for example, expectations concerning what people are like, but also affects the content of psychosis manifest in delusions, hallucinations, and social perceptions. Those who had experienced physical violence in their childhood tended to expect aggression or

DOI: 10.4324/9781003044956-8

violence both in everyday life and in psychotic states. Those with sexual abuse tended to be preoccupied by shame and contempt from others, again in both psychotic and non-psychotic beliefs and perceptions. Those who have been made refugees through political violence tended to have yearnings for that which was lost but also a fear concerning others. In spite of these potential links of meaning between the type of abuse and psychotic content, at least for those with child abuse, the connection between the past and present is not seen by the participant. This needs to be carefully considered in therapy.

Meaning generated in psychosis is a complex and evolving phenomena; possible influences include: the type of trauma, disturbance of motivations, the person's individual development, the person's family history and culture, and how the person engages in meaning-making, narration, and explanation. There is a transformation of meaning over time that involves continuities and alterations, the latter often obscuring the original meanings.

The participants reported what was described as extreme states of self and these included states of rage, dread, feeling inferior or defective, feeling distant, wanting control. It was also noted that in the experience of psychosis, and in particular persecution, there are transformations of what might be thought of as the identity of self and the perceived other. Often others are seen as some kind of attacking 'they' or alternatively an attacking semi-human entity. For some participants, at least for periods of time, there appears to be a psychotic transformation of the person's own identity, such as seeing oneself as a child or as a terrible killer. In terms of schema modes these can be thought of as psychoticised modes, parts, or states of self.

Our grasp of the everyday world requires a vast network of ideas we can access but also relies upon our dispositions to act in the world in a purposeful and skilful fashion. Psychotic experience implies not only a contradiction of ideas we might be able to articulate but also a suspension of dispositions that allow us to function in everyday contexts. The global set of dispositions to act in the world has been termed the background and includes what Wittgenstein described as bedrock certainties. Trust is part of our background in that we not only have certain explicit ideas about how or who to trust, and in what way to trust, but show this in our actions and dispositions.

Adults who suffer trauma such as torture have their background trust, certainties of everyday life, dispositions, and ways of living destroyed by the very process of trauma and emerge deeply changed. A person who has experienced abuse is likely to have a 'just about' coping or managing part of self, albeit with limitations, but also other disturbed and emotional parts, in particular, a self in terror. The latter and similar states operate without the full context of the background and usually contain extreme dispositions to mistrust.

Abuse and trauma lead to fear, anger, mistrust, but another common consequence is fluctuating depression. Most of the participants suffered episodes of depression to varying degrees. It was argued that depression involves 1) loss of a person's former pre-trauma 'lived identity', but also 2) a periodic loss of the 'just about' surviving self, the version of self that struggles in trying to recover from trauma and may, at least sometimes, keep depressive collapse at bay.

Abused children develop a coping part of self but also other parts which experience terror or anger. A child may manage developmental challenges throughout teenage years, but under the stress of new difficulties in adult years the terror self is reactivated and manifested. These parts of the self have a weak connection to background certainties of the everyday world. A terror part of the self will also contain implicit and explicit memories about the abusive adult, namely schemas of the other, and these schemas may be the basis for generating meaning found in hallucinations such as the words said or the character of the attacking entity. Abuse may also create epistemic mistrust which makes new learning difficult, in particular to discover that other people can be helpful, compassionate, and trustworthy.

The core argument concerning the generation of psychosis for adults or children is that trauma leads to many effects and these include loss of certainties and trust, fragmented parts of self, derealisation, existential feelings of threat and condemnation, negative meaning concerning self and others, negative emotion, and periodic depression. All these effects, to varying degrees, involve an alteration in foundational background capacities that connect a person to the shared everyday world, and without a firm connection to the background, psychotic ideas are generated and accepted as real.

Implications for therapy

The findings point to the potential importance of working with the effects of trauma for those with psychosis; however, it also suggests that caution is required in that clients are extremely unlikely to accept simple explanations and thematic links to the past. Furthermore, the person's experience of self and other has undergone profound changes and often these cannot be articulated by the client. The findings also point to the importance of trust, hope, the role of emotions, learning to cope with others, managing self states, and that such areas may be crucial for change.

Clearly the effects of trauma continue into the present and have colossal impact on the ability of individuals to live their lives. For some time therapists have explored whether, and in what way, therapy might be able to help those with psychosis and trauma. As will be seen, among these therapies there is a distinction between those which might directly address the trauma and ones which tend to work in a more indirect fashion, such as helping the person cope with emotions or social problems.

There have been several trials comparing the effect of using exposure, cognitive restructuring, Eye Movement Desensitisation and Reprocessing (EMDR), and imagery rescripting. The results tend to suggest that exposure and EMDR have some effect while cognitive restructuring itself was less effective (Steel, 2017). Work looking at imagery rescripting is a recent development in this area and is still being explored; I will return to this later. Exposure therapy involves clients attempting to remember details of the trauma and often to relive the experience with imagery. Cognitive restructuring involves challenging certain extreme negative meanings that may have occurred at the time of trauma, such as 'I will die'. EMDR involves a mixture of alternating sensory input, such as eye movements, and imagery.

Whether such therapies are effective or not, it is the case that many clients are extremely reluctant to approach any attempt at remembering a traumatic past. This can be difficult even when there is just one episode, such as an accident, but when abuse has continued for years then approaching these areas can be terrifying for clients. Van der Hart, Nijenhuis, and Steele (2006) in fact describe this as a phobia of traumatic memories. There may also be questions as to whether the very process of approaching such terrible memory is potentially harmful for some individuals. For these reasons several therapists, such as Rothschild (2017), have attempted to develop alternative methods of working with the effects of trauma; one general approach has been to work with sufferers of trauma to begin to cope with extreme emotions and to find strengths and resources to help them cope and reclaim their lives.

Indirect work for trauma and psychosis: constructional approaches

To work with psychosis and trauma in an indirect fashion, Rhodes and Jakes (2009) used a narrative approach drawing on aspects of narrative exposure therapy (Neuner et al., 2002) but also employed ideas from narrative and solution-focused therapies (de Shazer, 1988; White, 2007). The aim in this work was to set aside a small number of sessions and in those sessions to ask the client to tell the history of his or her life from before the trauma, during, and after. The clients were not asked to give details about specific trauma but to develop a narrative overview. The aim of the work was not 'exposure' to trauma or reliving. Where there seemed to be strong negative themes or idea about the self or events, the therapist commented upon this and sometimes explored alternative suggestions or explanations. There was also a strong focus on being constructional, that is, to articulate any ways of coping and find strengths, personal resources, or exceptions to the dominant negative narration. At the end of the work a letter was written to summarise what had been explored and read to the client in a session.

Other constructional approaches to trauma include the solution-focused work of Dolan (1991) with sexual abuse. Van der Kolk (2014) presents several therapies which aim to help the person develop strengths and well-being such as dance, singing, yoga, and therapies that focus on the expressive nature of the body. Two of these therapies he described are discussed below (sensorimotor therapy and internal family systems).

Concepts and therapies for the multiple self

Several therapies have at their core the idea that a person with extreme difficulties moves in and out of various extreme states of self, similar to the ways discussed in chapter six; some of these therapies have developed ways of working with individuals who have been abused or who have suffered other kinds of developmental difficulties. In the following I will give an outline of some of these therapeutic models. All these therapies involve helping the person understand and work with parts of the self and also to build up abilities to cope. I hope to show that one can draw on these therapies in helping clients who have psychosis as well as trauma. This selection is not a review of all the various possible therapies that use such concepts and there are approaches not covered here.

The mode concept in schema therapy

The concept of mode has become central to schema therapy (ST). Young, Klosko, and Weishaar (2003) state that a mode is 'those schemas or schema operations—adaptive or maladaptive—that are currently active for an individual'. A schema in general is defined as a broad pervasive theme or pattern composed of memories, emotions, cognitions, and bodily sensations (plus other features). Examples of modes include the categories of vulnerable child, detached protector, and critical parental mode. We can conceive a mode as consisting of a pattern of schemas which occur each time the mode is in operation. The degree to which a person is aware of having different modes varies with the individual. Young et al. note that the definition of mode is similar to the concept of 'states of mind' developed by Horowitz (1991).

Lazarus, Sened, and Rafaeli (2020) have researched how modes may manifest themselves over time. For this research they developed their own short-form mode questionnaire and recorded the following ten mode types: angry, distressed, self-critical, avoidant, perfectionist, self-soothing, compliant, contented, and self-reflective. They give as a description of modes: 'state-like manifestations of personality that function as cohesive organisational units. Such units possess distinct subjective qualities, and are characterised by specific affects, behaviours, cognitions, and desires that tend to be coactivated'. In contrast to Young, they did not specify that these states were specifically child or parental ones. ST uses a wide range of techniques including ones from CBT but also experiential methods such as imagery (Arntz & Jacob, 2013) and chair work. Details on the approach to trauma are given below.

Sensorimotor therapy

Fisher (2017) employs the structural disassociation model (SDM) of Van der Hart, Nijenhuis, and Steele (2006); however, she replaces the idea of 'apparently normal self' and instead suggests a 'going on with normal life personality', that is, a self that copes as best it can given the person's history of suffering. The 'going on with normal life' part is the one which just about manages in the context of daily life and functions well enough most of the time albeit imperfectly. She argues, following the SDM, that there is an 'emotional self' based on fundamental reactions such as fear, fight, freezing, and submitting, which have developed in the context of the person's life and trauma. Fisher emphasises the role of the body: how past and present suffering is both felt and demonstrated in the body.

A feature of Fisher's approach is to focus on the present experience of the person and in doing so to allow the person over time to become aware of their diverse states and sometimes to allow into consciousness experiences which have been dreaded and have rarely surfaced, such as a feeling of great distress. A key aim of Fisher's therapy is not to re-experience trauma, but to develop a sort of mindful awareness and a set of skills for grounding the person in the here and now. If a person, for example, expresses anxiety about a forthcoming social event, then she may work with that person to become aware that these are fears of a child part and to explore any implications of these fears. If a child part of the self fears humiliation, then the adult part can reassure the child part by saying that now, as an adult, 'I have the capacity to leave the party and not accept any insulting behaviour'. Often Fisher asks the person to return to being aware of feelings in the body. She also asks clients to check if there is felt to be some sort of unfinished action such as the urge to run away and then, if appropriate, to complete the action in the here and now.

Internal family systems

Schwartz (1995) developed Internal Family Systems (IFS) which describes three general types of state of self termed 'manager', 'exiles', and 'fire-fighters'. Exiles are those parts which might carry a person's distress and which the person often does not wish to acknowledge or tries to avoid. Firefighter parts will emerge to stop distress and take emergency action such as becoming drunk or engages in self-cutting. The manager parts of the personality are manifest most of the time and run the person's life, although at a cost of not being expressive, flexible, or open. While keeping in mind these three broad categories, Schwartz underlines the uniqueness of each person and the distinct manifestations of possible states of the self. The approach draws on a person's capacity to use imagery and metaphors. The parts are conceived as forming a group or a family and it is emphasised that any specific part will have relationships with other parts. The inter-part relations themselves might contribute to difficulties and this is often a focus of the therapy. In IFS it is not assumed that all parts are the product of trauma, rather, that it is the norm to have parts.

The dialogic and narrative self dialogue and parts of self

Lysaker and Lysaker (2001) developed therapy for psychosis employing the concept of the dialogic self (Herman & Dimaggio, 2004). The dialogic self conception is that a person is composed of many voices or 'I-positions' and that dialogues can occur between these positions; for example, one might speak from the point of view of being confident, but at other times, speak from a position of feeling vulnerable. The Lysakers noted that often narratives given by those with psychosis were minimal. One focus of therapy was to enrich the complexity of these positions and the narratives generated about the person's life. In recent work Lysaker and Klion (2018) have emphasised the practice of understanding the mental states of others and oneself.

Corstens, Longden, and May (2012) present a therapy for working with voices. A central aim is to explore the character and nature of the voices and how these emerged in the life of the person. There is careful attention to whatever difficulties and stresses the person might have experienced at the time of the onset and over time. There is an emphasis on developing, with the client, a narrative of the development of the voices. An important aspect of their work is to use the voice dialogue approach as developed by Stone and Stone (1989). Heriot-Maitland et al. (2019) expand the above describing how in therapy the character of different voices a person may have can be explored, and how compassion and motivational systems are relevant.

Overview of self-states theories

Clearly there are many theories and different conceptualisations of the states or parts of the self. Rowan (2010) reviewed many such theories spanning decades and argues that it is likely that there cannot be one definitive system of diverse parts of the self. In addition, there might be no one definitive conceptualisation of what exactly the parts are: for example, is a part just an extreme feeling or does it actually act as an autonomous personality with a will of its own? Whatever the validity of the different therapeutic systems, and even where we decide to use a particular model, it is still imperative that we approach each individual as unique and as having distinctive states of self.

In spite of the different theories and therapeutic practices, looking across the various theories it is apparent that similar types of self states are often suggested. Perhaps the most common of all is a version of a fearful or vulnerable self which may reflect difficult early experience. Another common state of self is one in which the person becomes critical and attacks the self. A third common state is being distant and detached from feelings or interaction with others. Versions of these three are found in most of the therapeutic models above. Also often suggested are states such as anger and the experience of shame or guilt. In chapter six the states that appeared in the three groups researched for this book were presented; several of these states of self overlap with the types given above.

Modified ST for psychosis?

Can ST be used for psychosis? And if yes, to what extent and in what ways? Originally, it had been suggested that clients with psychosis may not be suitable; however, with modifications and precautions I believe ST, and some related multi-self oriented therapies, can be used for individuals with psychosis. I will present illustrations of therapy I have carried out intended as preliminary investigations and note some research by others who have moved in this direction. While the main therapy I draw upon is ST, I will describe some selected ideas and techniques from other models of therapy in particular those in the above sections on the multi-self.

Rescripting

Several recent therapies have begun to explore the possibility of using imagery in the context of psychosis and have drawn on the approach of Arntz and Weertman (1999). Ison et al. (2014) reported work with four participants using imagery scripting. This involved a series of steps whereby the client both develops an image of themselves being comforted and supported by the therapist, and later where the client gives support and compassion to an image of the young self. The results suggest improvements in the experience of negative imagery. Paulick, Arnstz, and Steel (2019) reported a case-series of twelve participants with trauma and a diagnosis of psychosis. The main method of therapy was imagery scripting in stages, again the aim being to give comfort and support to the distressed child image. The results demonstrated a reduction in the voices, distress, frequency, and intrusions of trauma. Taylor et al. (2020) reported short-term therapy (assessment and then five sessions) with five participants who reported distressing imagery in the context of psychosis and persecutory delusions. Their work combined imagery rescripting and the cognitive behavioural approach of Hackman (2011). There was a focus on the person's negative schematic beliefs and negative imagery; one technique was to use transformation of the image by running the image on past the worst point or updating aspects of the image and sometimes using a connection to the past. They also used positive imagery of the future. The results suggested significant reductions in negative schemas, delusions, imagery distress, and changes in measures of schemas and schema modes.

Some preliminary cautions and guidelines for schema therapy with psychosis

The therapy reviewed above suggests that features of ST might be useful in working with psychosis and trauma. I wish now to present an approach that focuses on states of the self and moves towards a full use of ST. I have come to believe through clinical practice that either a partial or full use of ST and related therapies for states of self can be used for psychosis in general but also for psychosis with trauma given certain conditions and limits. In the following I outline some possible modifications and precautions.

It is still the case that ST will not be suitable for certain clients with psychosis, in particular, those who are in the midst of a crisis or show extreme psychotic thinking and perceptions such that any focus and collaboration would be extremely difficult. However, having a voice or paranoia or psychotic perception of others is not in itself, I believe, a barrier to therapy given that the person has consented to therapy, is motivated to attend, can sustain a focus, carry out homework, and to some extent is willing to talk about difficulties whatever these are.

One major precaution I believe is that there should be a concentration on immediate experience and in general an orientation to the here and now of the person. The starting point should be the experiential world of the client and what the person is suffering. There should not, therefore, be elaborate hypotheses or inferences going beyond the manifest surface or immediacy of experience; the latter being something that can be agreed upon by both the therapist and the client. If a client wishes to talk about a voice, then one should talk about the voice and how that entity affects the person; one would not at this stage of therapy make any inference about the origin or nature of the voice, or that the voice had come from abuse or trauma. A focus on trauma might in fact not be relevant at any stage for some clients. I believe it is essential that one stays 'in tune' with the person and respect their experiential lived world. Of course in the unfolding of therapy the dialogue will change in that the client may become more interested in alternative explanations and even ones focused on early years; however, they should only be explored when the person is clearly ready and is motivated to explore such topics.

Any linking to the past, at any stage of therapy, should only be done cautiously and presented as a tentative idea. When such topics were explored with participants in this book they did not link their psychotic experiences to abuse or trauma. I believe it is quite rare for clients to see this possibility. Of course to insist upon it would risk alienating the client; it might for example be seen as blaming the parents. For these reasons I do not think it useful with psychotic clients to present a full conceptualisation at the beginning of work; it is better to move to discussing such ideas over time and only as appropriate. In addition, any formulation should start in areas where there can be clear agreement, only slowly moving to other ideas and connections when the client seems open to such possibilities.

In line with the indirect approaches to trauma described above, I believe full exposure to trauma is unlikely to be accepted by clients, is probably not effective for complex trauma, and might in fact be retraumatising. It is also the case that some clients cannot remember what occurred; whatever produces this effect, for example, from motivation, from forgetting itself, or that memories were never formed in the first place, it remains that clients often only have limited access to explicit memory. Again, this points to the importance of working in the present moment.

As the work proceeds, and sometimes even at the beginning, a client might suggest a link to the past, or might doubt what a voice is, or if there is a plot; in general, I believe it is best not to assume that client has permanently cast aside any such extreme beliefs. Emersion in psychotic content is something that wavers; it is also the case that the person can apparently hold contradictory beliefs over extended time periods.

In general I have found the concept of state of self or mode as closer to the client's experience than the concept of 'schema'. The latter involves a certain amount of inference and theory; that is, one needs to explain that many diverse experiences indicate something underlying that produces the manifest experience. This in itself is difficult. It is also the case that many schema relate to trauma, developmental difficulties, and various very sensitive and upsetting issues such as not being cared for or feeling defective. For many psychotic clients these themes can be distressing, at least during early therapy and perhaps even much later. In general, therefore, in modifying ST for many clients I tend not to rely on explicit schema concepts; however, sometimes a specific schema theme with obvious supporting evidence can be useful (see below).

The therapeutic relationship might also need to be changed in working with psychosis. In ST for personality problems the therapist is very active in showing direct and explicit care for the person and often will comment on the relation itself. I believe in work for psychosis one needs to proceed slowly, to be open, friendly, and let the relation develop over time. The client will often have little or no trust in therapy or the psychiatric system. As chapter seven underlined, trust may be one of the most fundamental topics for psychosis and will be relevant to the therapeutic relationship. Trust can only be developed in small incremental steps over many sessions. One needs to give the client time and space to move nearer or further from the elements and process of therapy and in fact from the therapist: the client needs to retain a sense of control (as emphasised by Hermans, 1992, for all trauma therapy). Van der Hart and colleagues have written on the 'phobia of attachment' in trauma and how this affects establishing ther-apeutic rapport; this applies even more so in psychosis work.

Describing and accessing states of self

How can one assess and describe a person's multiple states of self? It is in fact quite natural to talk of a person as having different states: clients spontaneously say comments such as 'sometimes I am not myself', or 'part of me is very afraid'. In order to develop talk about such states the fol-lowing can be explored.

Direct questions for present and recent times

The simplest way is to note any strong feelings and reactions that have occurred in recent times, for example, with regard to hearing a voice or trying to travel on a bus, or in dealing with other people. As appropriate, one might explore the person's thoughts, feelings, bodily sensations, atti-tudes, and social interaction. One can then ask, 'is this a way of reacting you often experienced'? It is also useful to note how a client reacts and interacts while in assessment and how the person is with the therapist, for example, is a client relaxed and open, or somewhat closed and distant?

Further exploration of modes can involve asking a person to keep a structured diary of their states with questions on feelings, reactions, body state. For some clients at a later stage, the use of chairs can be helpful, that is, ask the person to sit in a chair and express how a critical part of self might express its thoughts.

Focus on types of situation

It can be useful to ask the person about how they feel in different situa-tions: for example, do aspects of the way you react concern you? Are you ever surprised by how you react in different situations? How would you list the different states you experience? Some specific questions are:

Do you criticise yourself? In what way?
Do you make a lot of demands on yourself? How do you speak to yourself? What do you say?

Do you ever feel cut off or with little feeling or emotion?

What is it like when you are most distressed, upset, lonely, despairing? What feelings do you have at such times?

Do you ever have anger or rage? What kind of situations does this happen in and what are you like at such times?

How do you behave and react in conflict with others?

Do you feel you are very different at different times? If so, in what way are you different at different times?

What is it like when you feel got at or attacked by others?

In addition to the above, one can take descriptions of modes given in ST or from the states of self as described by Fisher (2017) and discuss whether the client recognises any of these.

Using creative imagery

There are a range of interesting ideas for assessment presented by Schwartz which can, I believe, be combined with ST. In this approach if a particular state has been mentioned such as feeling angry, one might ask the client to imagine what that part might look like, adding that such an image might be of the person, or a transformation of the person, or that one could use the image of a character or symbol; for example, anger might well be represented by fire or an image of a red face and shaking fists. If an image of a part is formed, Schwartz suggests it is important to ask how the client feels towards that part; exploring anger, one could ask the client what they feel towards the anger image and here the person might say 'I feel afraid'. The client can be asked to place the anger image in a room and then move on to asking for an image of fear, and likewise explore how the client feels towards fear. This approach emphasises the relationships between parts. The technique is suitable for clients who are comfortable discussing their problems and find it easy to visualise; however, this is not the case for all.

Questionnaires

The Young Mode Questionnaire is complex yet all the clients with psychosis I have given this to have been willing to fill it in and were well able to understand the questions and give coherent answers. In general I have found this questionnaire to be very illuminating even if there are limitations, for example, on whether it covers all relevant modes for clients with psychosis. It is also useful to give the Young's Schema Questionnaire even if an in-depth investigation of schemas is not part of the work; first, it can help in understanding a client, and second, there are situations where one might just take one or two key themes and discuss these with the client in the context of exploring a mode state.

Upsetting situations and imagery

For clients who are very engaged in therapy and functioning well, one can draw directly on an assessment approach of Young, Klosko, and Weishaar (2003) whereby one would ask the client to visualise an upsetting childhood situation, usually with a caregiver, and explore how the person feels and what the person might need with regard to that adult figure. Unlike standard ST this might be something one attempts at a later stage in the work and not at the beginning.

Overview on assessment

Assessing the mode states of the person must be a joint endeavour; a state can only make sense if the client can access memories of what such a state feels like and that talking of it as a state makes sense to them. There should not be an imposition of theory or a sort of expert interpretation of something beyond given experience. This approach must stay close to what the person expresses. After a detailed assessment of states, it is useful to summarise the parts of self and present these to the client for feedback. One can also then ask which parts cause the person most concern and whether it might be helpful to alter how the state manifests itself.

Conceptualisation of William

Finally I wish in this chapter to present a brief conceptualisation of William, the case described in chapter five, showing how self states and other concepts in this book may cohere. The key features of William's childhood were that he did not know his biological mother, and subsequently was fostered with a couple who over years physically and

emotionally abused him. His delusional system focused on of being persecuted by a series of organisations including social services and terrorists.

In terms of core beliefs it was clear that he held extremely negative ideas
about himself; that he was, for example, bad or completely incapable. His
behaviour was generally one of withdrawing from the world and avoiding
social contact. His reactions and thoughts were focused on potential violence and threats from others; these meanings were manifest in his everyday thinking and emotions but also in psychotic content.

Besides the obvious fear he felt in the presence of his foster parents as a
child, his situation was incomprehensible: how could social services and his
foster parents abandon and abuse him yet these people were meant to care for
him? His mistreatment from a developmental perspective of course had an
impact on his emotions, style of attachment, and other basic human abilities
and needs, but also as a profound assault on the capacity to understand the
world, to know what is happening. He had memories of beatings and then
thinking whether he himself was to blame. Given Bill's experience of how
terrible and duplicitous the actions of his foster parents were, it is not surprising that he went on to form extreme mistrust of others.

In terms of mode states it was conspicuous that sometimes he felt rage
or that he felt vulnerable. In the presence of others he usually displayed
detachment. Of central importance was the mode of a terrified child self
who carried expectations or schemas of the other as attacking and untrustworthy, clearly based on the figures of his parents. It seems likely that
the terror state or vulnerable child part was not directly or fully accessible;
an aspect of his suffering was the mismatch of his adult self, who tried to
understand and cope, with the part of himself which was terrified and
generated images of attack.

Conclusion

There is a rich tradition of conceptualising psychosis as involving a fragmentation of the self and that this might be the product of a history of
trauma. Dating from at least Janet, it has also been theorised that the more
trauma has been experienced, the more likely it is that parts of the self are
not only disconnected but are disassociated such that the person in extreme
cases may not even be aware of their existence. There are now several
therapeutic approaches of working outside the constraints of directly

remembering and reliving traumatic events. In the next chapter I will illustrate therapy orientated towards imagery and the multi-self in the context of psychosis and trauma.

References

Arntz, A., & Jacob, G. (2013). *Schema therapy in practice*. Chichester: Wiley-Blackwell.

Arntz, A., & Weertman, A. (1999). Treatment of childhood memories: Theory and practice. *Behaviour Research and Therapy, 37*, 715–740.

Corstens, D., Longden, E., & May, R. (2012). Talking with voices: Exploring what is expressed by the voices people hear. *Psychosis, 4*, 95–101.

de Shazer, S. (1988). *Clues: Investigating solutions in brief therapy*. New York: Norton.

Dolan, Y.M. (1991). *Resolving sexual abuse: Solution-focused therapy and Ericksonian hypnosis for adult survivors*. New York: Norton

Fisher, J. (2017). *Healing the fragmented selves of trauma survivors*. New York: Routledge.

Hackman, A. (2011). Imagery rescripting in posttraumatic stress disorder. *Cognitive and Behavioral Practice, 18*, 424–432.

Heriot-Maitland, C., McCarthy-Jones, S., Longden, E., & Gilbert, P. (2019). Compassion focused approaches to working with distressing voices. *Frontiers in Psychology, 10*, 152. 10.3389/fpsyg.2019.00152

Herman, J.L. (1992). *Trauma and recovery*. New York: Basic Books.

Herman, J.M., & Dimaggio, G. (eds.) (2004). *The dialogical self in psychotherapy*. London: Routledge.

Horowitz, M.J. (1991). Person schemas. In M. Horowitz (ed.), *Person schemas and maladaptive interpersonal patterns* (pp. 13–32). Chicago: University of Chicago Press.

Ison, R., Medoro, L., Keen, N., & Kuipers, E. (2014). The use of rescripting imagery for people with psychosis who hear voices. *Behavioural and Cognitive Psychotherapy, 42*, 129.

Lazarus, G., Sened, H., & Rafaeli, E. (2020). Subjectifying the personality state: Theoretical underpinnings and an empirical example. *European Journal of Personality. 34*(6), 1017–1036. 10.1002/per.2278.

Lysaker, P.H., & Lysaker, J.T. (2001). Psychosis and the disintegration of dialogical self-structure: Problems posed by schizophrenia for the maintenance of dialogue. *British Journal of Medical Psychology, 74*, 23–33.

Lysaker P.H., & Klion R.E. (2018). *Recovery, meaning-making, and severe mental illness: a comprehensive guide to metacognitive reflection and insight therapy.* Abingdon-on-Thames: Routledge.

Neuner, F., Schauer, M., Roth, W.T., & Elbert, T. (2002). A narrative exposure treatment as intervention in a refugee camp: A case report. *Behavioural and Cognitive Psychotherapy, 30,* 205–209.

Paulik, G., Steel, C., & Arntz, A. (2019). Imagery rescripting for the treatment of trauma in voice hearers: A case series. *Behavioural and Cognitive Psychotherapy, 47,* 709–725.

Rhodes, J., & Jakes, S. (2009). *Narrative CBT for psychosis.* Hove: Routledge.

Rothschild, B. (2017). The body remembers. Vol 2. *Revolutionizing trauma treatment,* London: Norton.

Rowan, J. (2010). *Personification.* London: Routledge.

Schwartz, R.C. (1995). *Internal family systems therapy.* New York: Guilford.

Steel, C. (2017). Psychological interventions for working with trauma and distressing voices: The future is in the past. *Frontiers in Psychology, 7,* 2035. doi: 10.3389/fpsyg.2016.02035

Stone, H., & Stone, S. (1989). *Embracing our selves: The voice dialogue manual.* Novato: New World Library.

Taylor, C., Bee, P., Kelly, J., Emsley, R., & Haddock, G. (2020). iMAgery focused psychological therapy for persecutory delusions in PSychosis (iMAPS): A multiple baseline experimental case series. *Behavioural & Cognitive Psychotherapy, 48,* 530–543.

Van der Hart, O., Niejenhuis, E., & Steele, K. (2006). *The haunted self: Structural dissociation and the treatment of chronic traumatisation.* New York, USA: Norton.

Van der Kolk, B.A. (2014). *The body keeps the score: Brain, mind and body in the healing of trauma.* New York: Viking Press.

White, M. (2007). *Maps of narrative practice.* New York: Norton.

Young, E., Klosko, J.S., & Weishaar, M.E. (2003). *Schema therapy: A practitioner's guide.* New York: Guilford Press.

9

DIALOGUE AND IMAGERY WITH STATES OF SELF

This chapter will illustrate how a modified form of schema therapy (ST) can be employed for those with psychosis and histories of abuse. The following sorts of work are described: assessment; how one can help clients with emotional and social problems; coping with symptoms such as voices or paranoia; and how to approach the effects of trauma. The chapter concludes with a detailed case presentation. The chapter is not intended as a full outline of how such therapy might be carried out. The case illustrations are reconstructed from different clients with details altered to preserve anonymity.

Assessment and phases of therapy

It is useful to plan therapy as a sequence of stages in line with those therapies specifically aimed at trauma (Van der Hart, Niejenhuis & Steele, 2006). Therapy will normally start with assessment and then move on to helping the client achieve stability in the present, that is, to try to sort out

DOI: 10.4324/9781003044956-9

any pressing concerns and make sure the client is engaging in any of the positive ways of coping already known to the client but not being used. Once a client has achieved some sort of stability, and a working therapeutic relationship is established, work can focus on the effects of modes in the daily life of the person, such as how he or she might engage in self-criticism. Next it can be useful to look at the symptoms themselves and how the client can change them or better cope. If a client is in agreement, and there is need, a next major phase can be one of looking at the effects of trauma. A final phase is usually helping the client to reclaim their life in various ways by making social changes and taking up a wider range of activities concerning interests or work. Of course with psychosis the therapist must always be maximally flexible; if a client is in crisis, then attention should be on helping the client get through the crisis with a strong focus on how to cope and survive the present situation.

I will not attempt in this chapter a full account of how to assess clients; this will depend on the client and the details of the therapy used. How to assess states of self or modes was outlined in chapter eight; such assessment might take place at the beginning of therapy, but might be returned to at any stage. Several ideas on assessment in phases and the approaches used for the clients in this chapter are described in Rhodes and Jakes (2009). Details on formulation will not be given in this chapter.

Working with modes for persistent emotional and social problems

In this section I will look at therapy using modes focused on emotional and social difficulties and not symptoms or trauma. Different types of mode state tend to be treated in different ways. For the vulnerable or child part the aim will be to give care, support, and compassion; in contrast, work with a critical part of the self aims to stop the attacks upon the person. Following ST, but also internal family systems (IFS) of Schwartz (1995), it is assumed that various mode states can be protective for the person, even if they tend to lead to difficulties such as when a child may has learnt to be compliant with others in order to survive. In this section I will describe working with the states of being compliant, critical, angry, and vulnerable. For all the below-mentioned mode states, the part will be relevant when its role is manifest in a social or emotional problem; for example, the person is afraid of going to the shops due to excessive fear, or the person feels demoralised and frustrated due to being too kind to others.

Vulnerable self

The aim is to develop a picture of the part of the self that is vulnerable and then to give comfort and express care to that vulnerable self. This can be done in a variety of ways using mental imagery and dialogues; for example, the person can imagine talking to the vulnerable self saying caring and reassuring things. Alternatively, the client can visualise someone who they find to be caring and speak to that person, or create an image of the caring person embracing and holding them. Some clients, of course, find this very difficult and such work has to be built up cautiously, often modelled first by the therapist. Examples are given below from therapy with Adrian, Greg, and Susan.

Critical self

During the assessment, or later, the person might begin to see how they are critical of themselves; often this needs careful discussion since the person believes it is either normal or justified. The therapist may need to outline how excessive criticism can lead to demotivation and distress. In ST the idea in general is to stop the critical self. For example, one could suggest not listening to this part and trying to ignore its more extreme comments. Often chair work is used; clients talk in the voice of the attacker, but then move to another chair to respond from a caring perspective. The therapist and client address the punitive mode stating that what it says is not acceptable.

The approach of IFS is somewhat different; the person strikes up a dialogue in imagery with the critical part and asks a series of questions: Do you know what you do to the client? Do you know the effect of doing that? What do you think would happen if you stopped doing that, for example, being so harsh? If the critical part makes a comment such as 'if I don't criticise then he will be weak', then one can ask how the client might achieve not being 'weak' so the critical part stops its attacks. The emphasis in IFT is not a rejection of the attacking part but an attempt to change how it functions in the life of the person. The critical part is then told that the adult self will look after these things and does not require such extreme commentary.

Adrian

Adrian stated in the assessment that he was critical all the time and made comments such as 'I've not done enough', 'I need to do more', and then yet more negative comments such as 'I should die' or 'give up' and 'I'm useless', and that he was never going to be anything. Asking for the most extreme sorts of comments he said, 'I'm a f*****g idiot'. For such extremity of self attack much work is needed to help the person try to be self compassionate (details of therapy with Adrian are given in later sections). If IFS was used, one would ask what would happen if this part stopped such insults, and linked to this, how the client would need to change. The critical parts of those abused are often extremely powerful and many sessions and approaches are needed to create change.

Angry self

Using mode therapy one can ask the person to express anger, and sometimes to do this by sitting on a different chair and speaking from that mode. The aim of the work is to allow an expression of anger yet to find ways that are not destructive. The very act of thinking about one's anger puts distance between the angry part and taking action. Accessing the more rational and compassionate part tends to have an effect of calming anger and making thought more flexible.

With the IFS technique one can ask the client to imagine the angry part of oneself, and if possible to actually see it and share this description. Therapy proceeds by asking why this part is so angry and what does it really wish for the client. The client can then say to the angry part that it will deal with these things in a reasonable and considerate fashion but the adult self will not forget the basic things that the anger part is concern about. Anger is often felt when the person is not standing up for themselves; under those circumstances, the client often needs help with being more assertive.

Luke

For Luke anger was a frequent problem when walking by other men on the street. He was asked for an image of this anger state and gave a picture of someone with clenched fists and a red aggressive face. When asked what he felt towards this part of self he described feeling fear that it was so extreme but also felt that the aggressive part was strong. When the image of anger was asked about its role in Luke's life it said that it protected him. Asked if there would be any negative consequences if it stopped being so extreme the reply was that Luke might be attacked by others. When asked how Luke could behave so that the anger part did not need to be so extreme when on the street it said that Luke would have to show more self-confidence by walking at a calm pace, looking around but not staring at others, and remembering he still had his strength and anger if really needed. Luke said he might be able to do these things and attempted to put them into practice.

Compliant self

Some clients often put themselves in a powerless position of always doing what others want or never expressing a preference. One can discuss with the client the advantages and disadvantages of this way of interacting and explore what an alternative and preferred way of acting might look like. Here the aim is to build up a person's strengths and confidence and to envisage how to behave in new ways.

Greg

When asked for a word or phrase to describe behaving in a compliant way Greg said, 'a pushover'. He was able to articulate that he did far too much for others, but if he did not do these things, he tended to feel he had been 'terrible'. He then mentioned that when he hadn't been compliant, he had often regarded himself as 'mean' and engaged in self-criticism. In therapy he was able to note how being compliant was linked to being bullied by his father as a child and that it had been a way of surviving. Working on intrusive self-criticism, and comforting the vulnerable child, allowed Greg to start experimenting with being more assertive (see further details on Greg in the trauma section).

Working with modes and psychotic symptoms
Paranoia and caring for the terrified self

For clients with psychosis and trauma, often their suffering most clearly manifests itself in everyday situations that in various ways relate to specific voices or delusions. Adrian had developed a very complex persecutory set of ideas concerning a secret organisation and usually thought that whenever he went to a place, such as the local shops or gym, that this was where he would be attacked or that something terrible but unspecified would happen. With careful investigation one usually finds that as clients enter the relevant daily situation they have extreme reactions of fear or panic and confused thought. Furthermore, they may experience an increase in the frequency or ferocity of their voices and their actual perception of others can alter. In such situations the client is probably entering into a state of child-related terror, as described in chapter six, though other fears might have different origins, such as adult experiences of abuse or mistreatments. The details, and how they are manifested, differ for each client and in therapy there is a need to map the states individually.

Given a client has expressed a wish to return somewhere, Adrian wanted to go back to the gym, then one can begin to work with the person to develop being calm, find ways of coping, and invite the person to practice these techniques in the difficult situation. A powerful addition here, with clients who are ready, is to fully engage in a conversation about how this terrified part of the self is exactly the same sort of feeling and state that that person experienced during trauma and abuse. One can therefore say to such a client: when you go into that situation you are re-experiencing the terrors that you underwent as a child and you need to calm those fears and look after that part of yourself.

Of course it would appear that such a set of ideas directly contradicts the claims made in the paranoid plot. However, I have found in therapeutic practice that one can simply engage in this way of talking without spelling out or discussing any contradictions. Rather it is useful to leave the truth of the issue open. Sometimes the contradiction does not become an issue: that is, one might talk about the plot, but on other occasions one talks about the person's fears and how to cope with these. Of course it is useful that the person does acknowledge the contribution of the past and directly sees that connection; however, working this way is possible even if the person has a fluctuating conviction in their persecutory ideas, and many clients are like this.

There are several ways of carrying out such work: with some clients it may be useful to use imagery whereby they imagine going into that difficult situation and then engage in self-talk and directly calm the self; techniques such as deep breathing and muscle relaxation are very helpful. There are also other ideas developed in body-orientated therapy (Fisher, 2017), for example, not only talking to a part as one enters the situation but moving the body, standing upright and then focusing on how this feels.

Adrian and paranoia

When asked at an early stage about what his paranoia felt like he said that 'they' were trying to kill him, to read his mind. He felt sometimes that the end of the world was coming or that something bad was going to happen. Adrian also heard voices and these contributed to his fear. At a later stage in the work he was asked what it would be like to be in the park, somewhere he wanted to visit: he said that he would feel scared and ask himself, 'why am I here'?; he would be afraid that he looked like a 'weirdo' and perhaps they would video him on mobile phones; he would be sure that something bad would happen. In continuing to explore his fears, he said that in the park they might record him on CCTV and then send him to jail. We were then able to begin to think how he could comfort and look after the vulnerable part of himself. He began to remind himself that nothing had happened in the past and that he had committed no crime. I was also able to have a discussion with him about the fact that if the persecutory or-ganisation was going to harm him they could have done it long ago.

In the next phase of work we developed his ability to be compassionate to himself; he learnt to answer the thought, 'I'm being lazy', with the thought, 'at least I'm trying'. We did a series of imagery work: first, he spoke about how not moving forward in his life was his fault, but he was then able to say things would work out. Next, he formed an image of the paranoid part which was rocking to and fro. He asked the image, 'what's wrong?' and the paranoid part replied that the Organisation was planning something. I encouraged Adrian then to speak to this paranoid part and he managed to say: 'don't worry, they are not out to get you... it will be fine... you've lived with this for years and nothing bad has happened... it will be fine... it just looks unsure... listen, I know how to handle things'. Adrian had also learnt in other sessions how to use deep breathing and muscle relaxation; he was encouraged to apply these in the situation. Though very difficult, and at first with the help of family members, he eventually started doing more activities, including going to the gym.

Adrian had severe difficulties and a full range of psychotic symptoms; in terms of being convinced that persecution was taking place, his levels were very high. Clients with less psychopathology are able to more openly contemplate the hypothesis of a child part and its influence; this was mentioned to Adrian but was something he found difficult. According to the stage of work, and the level of the client, different ways of framing the problem can be developed and used by the client in the terrifying context; for example, some clients are well able to begin to say to themselves that they know that this part is triggered by situations in the present but in fact the fear comes from the past. They can tell themselves that nothing is happening and that this is just the old fear, and coupled with this, engage in direct calming of the self and body.

Building the rational and compassionate self: alternative perspectives on paranoia

At some stages of therapy with some clients one can have a very open discussion about the contrast of two different ways of looking at something: typically, one is a fearful and persecutory perspective, and the other might well be a rational and compassionate one. One technique here is to use chair work; the person might be invited to sit in one chair and fully articulate all fears about what they think might be happening, what they might think when in a frightening situation. In the other chair the client can be invited to articulate the alternative perspective; this can range from simple comforting and compassionate words to a rational and evidence-based alternative. It is a conventional approach in cognitive therapy with delusions to sometimes consider contradictory evidence or inconsistencies; using chair work facilitates the client to have a self-generated internal dialogue and can help the therapist avoid slipping into the position of someone trying to persuade the client.

Adrian and chair work

At a later stage of work, Adrian was able to sit in one chair and express his dreads. He said: 'I feel fear… people are trying to record a crime and set me up and they may also poison my drinks'. He then sat in another chair and said: 'but no one is trying to kill you, the police aren't concerned and we've been through this before'. Encouraged to speak to the most fearful part he then said: 'how do you know?...you don't know the future'. The fearful part replied: 'but the Organisation are really powerful, you need to be scared'. In the other chair he was then able to say: 'if they need to kill me they would have done it by now... It's implausible... And how could anyone read my mind?' In this session he was also able to at least consider the possibility that some experiences might have their origin in psychosis. Using chairs for alternative perspectives and work on comforting the vulnerable self can build on each other. As stated, the degree to which the work might involve an open challenging of delusional ideas, as opposed to a more pure focus on reassurance and compassion, will depend on each client.

Working with voices

Hallucinatory voices can also be explored using imagery, chair work, and modes. Adrian was hearing very negative voices over many months. He said that they occurred on most days and made doing activities very difficult; they abused him and called him useless. Adrian was asked to form a visual image of the people who were generating voices: he said that one was a male social worker and the other was a woman using a microphone; he thought they were in a room somewhere and were watching a screen. He imagined that they were laughing at him, for example, for being overweight. I asked how he felt towards them and he said that he had a sense of 'mystery of what was reality' and questioned how 'the world worked'. When I asked again he then said he felt 'neutral' to the voices and I asked for an image of the part that felt neutral: he said that this part had 'wide eyes', looked shocked, and said that the world was 'crazy' and that he was afraid of the future. However, when further asked how he felt at other times, he said there was also an angry part; when asked how he saw this part he said it had an angry face and was upset and was 'someone who needed a break'. Then, when asked how he felt towards the angry part he said he felt calm, though he did feel a little sad as well. When that was explored, he said he felt 'friendly' to the sad part. Schwartz (1995) suggests that by asking such a sequence of questions sometimes one arrives at a more compassionate attitude or at least one of simple curiosity; this is an important step towards the self accepting different parts. The questions here showed that he had complex reactions to the voices, including at least puzzlement, anger, and sadness.

Returning to this work in another session, when he was hearing the voice calling him 'stupid', we used chair work. From one chair he spoke as the voice saying: 'I told you he is weird' expressed with laughter and a sneer. Adrian was then invited to speak from another chair and here to take a compassionate and more rational perspective. He stated to the voice about himself: 'he's not stupid and he's not going to give you power, he doesn't have a full psychiatric illness, he is smart you're failing to influence him'. Sitting in the voice chair he reported the voice as saying: 'aha you're an idiot, you will never do something with your life', that is, the voice-part continued to be negative. The work continued with an image of the vulnerable child part being helped and given assistance; the adult part was able to say that he would work to get rid of the voices. He was also able to say that he would not let the voices stop him and he would go shopping and go to the gym. The imagery suggested that the voices intimidated the child part of Adrian and an important feature of the work was to develop a more compassionate, caring, and rational attitude to the fears of the terrified child self and this focus continued throughout the rest of the work allowing him to return to public places.

Working with trauma and psychosis

Once there has been progress in helping the client make changes in their lives, and a working therapeutic relationship is well established, for some clients it may be appropriate to work with the meaning and effects of trauma. This clearly must be something the client is fully committed to and which makes sense to the client. In chapter eight several approaches were described for trauma or where there is both trauma and psychosis; some of these might be useful in combination with mode focused therapies, for example, using a narrative approach as in Rhodes and Jakes (2009). In this section I will explore therapy focused on states of self.

ST and IFS have developed approaches not only aimed at working with the diverse parts of the self but both have developed specific ways of working with trauma. For most clients with psychosis and abuse, I find that the phase of giving support and compassion to the child image to be a key therapeutic task. Where possible, the image of the client's adult caring self should be involved, but this can present great challenges. In this section I shall give an outline of these two potential approaches and give one brief and one longer case presentation.

Hayes and Wijngaart (2020) describe a series of steps used in ST for difficult and traumatic memories; in the first stage a client remembers a difficult episode but does not include the details of the traumatic events. It is suggested that the therapist should then intervene in the imagery, as any good caring adults would, to give compassion, aide, and care to the trouble child. This first stage therefore is one where the therapist carries out active imagery work in supporting the vulnerable child. In a second stage the client is more active. The therapy here uses a series of techniques described by Arntz and Weertman (1999): 1) the image is set up with the client as a child; 2) the client comes into the image as their adult self and supports and takes care of the child, stopping any mistreatment; 3) the client experiences the situation from a child's perspective and experiences being cared for by a visualisation of their adult self. Hayes and Wijngaart emphasise the importance of dealing with what they term the 'antagonist', that is the demanding or abusing parent or other figure.

A major aim of IFS is to get to know a person's parts usually using imagery: for example, there might be work in developing a characterisation of a critic part and then negotiating with that part so it becomes less attacking, and if possible, to find a new role such as giving helpful advice. After some progress, and when the client is ready, work focused specifically on trauma might be initiated. For trauma, they suggest the following steps: 1) a child self is imagined in a situation of potential abuse or trauma, 2) the child image is asked to show what is needed, so that the adult self and the therapist can understand, and what would be sufficient in order for the child to feel that it can leave this episode of life behind, and 3) once this is complete, the adult self enters and does whatever a responsible and caring adult would do in such a situation. The adult asks the child part if there is anything else that it wants doing before it is ready to leave. Later work invites the child part to come to the present or a safe place and to be present with the adult self. I find that drawing on specific techniques of IFS in an ST framework works well for some clients, particularly those with vivid visual imagination; other clients seem either less able to generate images or just feel uncomfortable using this approach. For the latter clients, dialogue work and simple images from memory seem more acceptable. I have also found the IFS method helpful in some cases of less extreme abuse and in doing short-term work.

Greg: abusive father and attacking voice

Greg experienced a repetitive negative voice; I explored the sorts of things it said and the tone of voice. I asked where he thought this voice came from. Greg thought that it was similar to the voice he used to hear from his father. In one session he said that the voice was calling him 'evil' and that this way of talking, or rather shouting, was like his father. Coping with this voice required many pieces of work. One was to access how he felt in the presence of this voice; this led to the experience of a terrified child part. Next, the major focus was to find ways of giving compassion to that part.

Using imagery I was able to help the child get away from the situation and to show how a caring adult would act and speak to such a child, that is, to give compassion, care, and to take protective action such as removing the child from harm. This approach is one recommended in ST for supporting the vulnerable child mode. Greg often made very negative comments about himself (i.e., from a 'punitive parent' mode). On several occasions I was able to talk to the distressed part in a compassionate way. Greg was able to practice this using chairs and he did homework in the form of self-talk.

When asked if anyone had ever helped him as a child, Greg was able to remember a caring uncle. Recruiting this possible resource, Greg was asked to remember this good person, how he would speak, and how he intervened to stop abuse when he could; Greg was then able to imagine this person speaking and giving comfort to him in the present.

We also used imagery so that Greg could learn to stand up to the abusive figure; he imagined his father being put away behind a metal barrier. On another occasion we were able to imagine the father sitting on a chair before us and I was able to tell him how I thought his behaviour had been terrible but also weak. Greg practiced in imagery how he, now as a grown man, would speak and stand up to his father. In general, the work over time consisted in caring for the child part, coming to understand the injustice of his abuse, and standing up to the negative image of an attacking father. It was also important to work on how Greg tended to blame himself for past events and how he continued to engage in extreme self-attacking statements. At one moment the image of the father was shouting at Greg; I was able to help Greg remember that now his father was no longer alive. Like Susan below, it is almost as if on some occasions the person has forgotten that someone is dead, or rather, moves in and out of any certainty they may have concerning a final disappearance of the abusing other. It may be that these fluctuations and uncertainty stem from the fact that a child part still believes the 'attacker' is alive.

Introduction to Susan

Susan had the same level of terrible emotional and physical abuse as Greg, but unlike him, did not seem to have any other caring person in the family. The degree and extent of Susan's psychosis were extreme and long-standing. Many therapeutic ideas were put in practice but a core focus was giving supportive statements and attempting to give care to the image of a child self. However, to allow any sort of image of her young self to come into consciousness, distant or faint, was difficult and took many months. For Susan I was not able, as the therapist, to model in imagery giving care since she only started to generate images after several weeks and at first always at home; furthermore, she found trust and the acceptance of care from others to be very difficult, and so even at a later stage still turned down this possibility.

Susan

Susan was a 40-year-old woman who had suffered for many years intrusive and aggressive voices. When I met her there was no obvious prolonged delusions though during our work she suggested that there may be a plot to kill her at that time, and that she sometimes thought she was the cause of some terrible events in the world. Susan suffered from repeated episodes of depression and over several years had engaged in forms of self-harm such as hitting herself on the head. She was, however, someone well engaged in community activities: she worked for a local charity helping to run activities with others and was connected to her local church. She had two friends who she would see occasionally. She lived alone and had had no relationship for several years. I had the impression that she was well engaged in therapy though reserved and cautious; she was rarely emotional in the sessions, in spite of the difficult topics addressed. Her ability to speak and think seemed clear. In terms of her childhood she reported great difficulties and abuse: her father had frequently used physical violence against her. Furthermore, her mother did not protect her nor seemed concerned by what was occurring. Her parents were not warm or affectionate towards her and in fact were often rejecting or critical. She had not received any type of psychotherapy as a child or adult.

The first sessions were basic assessments in which the aim was to explore the details, as reported above, to begin a basic working relationship, and to decide together what to focus on. When asked for her goals, Susan said: to stop the self-harm, in particular, hitting her head; to achieve forgiveness for her father and 'let it go'; to forgive herself for being 'a fool' and being 'promiscuous'; and to change the anger she felt towards herself. When asked what were the most important of these things she gave in order: being able to stop the self-harming, to forgive her father and to help cope with her voices.

The therapy involved many elements carried out at different stages and included: assessment and planning; resources and solution-orientated work; a narrative phase looking at the history of abuse and its effects; work on self-esteem; a focus on being compassionate and supportive to herself using imagery and dialogues; and at several states, developing a conceptualisation. In short, this was in part the approach described in Rhodes and Jakes (2009) then moving on to a modified version of ST.

Solution-orientated work

After the initial assessment, the first phase of work used solution-focused questions such as asking what tends to limit or stop self-cutting, what works with the voices, what goals she wanted to realise, when the problems were less or not occurring, how she would recognise change, and the use of the future-focused question, that is, a description of life without the problems. She was able to articulate the following strategies: she could, when distressed, listen to music, engage in drawing, read the Bible, not stay in bed when feeling depressed, and visit her chapel. Perhaps most important for her was that we articulated a notion of some behaviours being in line with what the 'devil' would require of her and some being what 'Jesus' or 'God' would encourage; in this I was using the conceptual framework she herself provided. She reminded herself that she was able to ask the question: 'should I follow the Devil's way or God's way?' The idea that to self-harm was in fact not in line with her religious beliefs came completely from Susan. In therapy I was therefore able to think with her what the implications of such beliefs might be. I also noted with her that one of her resources was that she was kind and generous; to such ideas she would listen but not give any sign of agreement. Having articulated the above list we went back to the ideas of coping at many stages of therapy, particularly whenever she was more stressed or upset.

Narrative and first imagery exploration

By the tenth session we decided to focus on trauma. For this work my aim was to draw on the approach described in Rhodes and Jakes (2009), which involves constructing a narrative with the person giving an overview of both negative and positive events without reliving. Susan, however, could remember extremely little of what had occurred during her childhood. There were, nevertheless, some quite disturbing specific memories, such as that her father had boasted that he began to slap her even while she had been a young baby. One vivid memory was that at six years of age she thought that she was going to die. When not hitting her he tended to be critical and usually distant or out of the house working. When he became angry she said he became a 'monster' and that she thought he was 'used by the devil'. At the age of nine she remembered wishing that he was dead. When he had actually died many years later, she remembered thinking at the graveside that he was still alive. And it turned out that in fact she often had the thought that he might still be alive.

One part of our work was to review the fact that he was dead and she could, between sessions, remind herself of this reality. When I asked her how she felt concerning her memories she replied: 'I feel revolted', that her heart felt as 'water in a storm', and she felt anger and fear. She then added that it was 'like a knife cutting inside me'. Clearly this is a terrible mixture and turmoil of reactions. I worked immediately trying to find an image of peace. In the next session she said she had blotted out most memories, but had had negative thoughts about herself, in particular, one of blaming the child she had been. Here I made my first attempt at working with a child image of Susan; however, she could not get an image from memory or imagination, so I asked her to just listen to me addressing that part, giving support, and telling that part she was not to blame. In several therapies using imagery there is the recommendation that the therapists model in imagery the giving of care to a child self; this was not possible with Susan at any stage as stated above.

During this phase she was able to use imagery concerning her father. When she tried to imagine him she said that she felt great fear and was not able to directly speak to him or tell him to back off or go away. In the end what worked was for her to imagine a picture of Jesus who was able to make her father disappear into 'black smoke'. She was very relieved that she could imagine this and mentioned in a later session that she had done this several times by herself. We revised the idea that her father was now dead and she said she would keep reminding herself of this during the following weeks.

The investigation of the past revealed several key features, in particular that she regarded herself as somehow 'bad' (she gave as evidence for this that she had sex with some boyfriends during her teens), and, as stated, that sometimes she had the idea that her father was still alive though knowing that he was dead. In terms of positive narrative, I noted first how she had changed her life and found a stable home, how she was helpful and kind to others and made tentative suggestions that some of the episodes of her adult life, where she blamed herself for what had happen, might have followed as a consequence of her suffering and low self-esteem.

Self-esteem and compassion work

In the next phase of work the idea of being kind or compassionate to oneself was explained and Susan was given sheets to take home, whereby she could record her negative self-attacking thoughts, and then, in contrast, think of what a kind or compassionate thought would be. This work drew on the ideas of compassion therapy as developed by Gilbert (2010). She was very good at attempting this homework though she found it very difficult. We also used the idea of looking for evidence of positive features about oneself, and looking at evidence over time of what made her think she was good or bad (Padesky, 1994).

For some negative thoughts she was able in writing to give a few tentative compassionate alternatives. On one sheet she had written that her feeling was of a need to cut herself; as an alternative she wrote 'the little girl said to me "don't hurt me"…why should I do to myself what my parents did to me'? (See the next section for how this image of a girl was relevant and how it developed.)

When she was attacking herself for being 'fat' (as she wrote) she was able to say in the compassionate column of the form that God had created her body and that she should not worry since she would have a heavenly body. She was also able to simply reject some of the negative claims, for example, by stating that she was not 'fat' and that she was not responsible for the deaths of children in a recent terrorist attack. This negative belief suddenly emerged in our work; I suspect, however, that she had had many versions of this sort of idea and with delusional intensity.

Working with imagery and the child self

The aim of this work was to articulate with Susan various 'parts' or modes of herself and consider how she related to these parts. This work borrowed from ST but unlike ST did not make explicit detailed links between recent episodes and past events. At several points, particularly later in the work, the idea of her present suffering being related to her early years and mistreatment were suggested. Parallels between the particular nature of her voice and the mistreatment she experienced were also discussed; this, however, was completely open and presented as just possibilities. At this stage she could at least consider an alternative narrative to what she was undergoing. As discussed earlier, it seems possible there can be interest by a client in two very different explanations or narratives.

A particular focus was to consider the vulnerable part of herself and the person she was as a child. We attempted again to construct an image of the young Susan; the idea being that we would think of some way of imagining giving care to that younger self. However this continued to be very difficult. At first Susan could still get no image whatsoever of little Susan. We noted together how this was the case and how difficult this task was. Over several weeks, however, she was eventually able to form a basic image of a young self between sessions. She told me that at first the image of Susan would stay at a great distance and even cower from her. One step forward was in reviewing her teenage years and her rebellious behaviour; to this image she still could not be supportive but did manage to say 'I understand you'.

Eventually, in one session she reported getting an image of her young self that was 'like a moving picture'. I suggested she could touch or hold little Susan, but Susan reported that the young self 'winced' and 'cowered'. I wondered whether she could say that she didn't want to harm the child. Susan said that this was difficult 'because I am a bad person'. I asked if she wished to harm the child, if she would do that if she could, and she said no. I emphasised the importance of that; she was then able to make contact between the adult and child, the image being of just touching the tips of each others' fingers. The child smiled and Susan said the child self was then playing. From this time on using imagery slowly became easier, though with some setbacks; it required continuous encouragement and affirmation that she was not aiming to harm the child and that she was not a bad person. We returned to being kind to the child image many times during the following sessions and it was suggested the child and adult could attempt to hold hands. In one later session the child image said: 'he is coming to hit me' but Susan got rid of this threat and told the child image that 'he's gone... I will protect you... we are together'.

In another piece of imagery work she was asked to imagine the attacking-hallucinated voice. During the assessment she had said that this voice was like a 'black fist'; she further explained that she thought the voice was trying to make her kill herself so she would go to hell. In one session, to help her cope with the voice, I asked her to visualise what the voice might look like at that moment. She said she saw it like a blade trying to cut her. I asked how she could cope with this image, or how she could change the image; she was able to imagine a wave of light which would dismiss the blade and which would protect her. She also said to the image of the blade that it was not going to harm her.

Together at one point we summarised what appeared to be the main parts or states of Susan: these were 'detached', the 'self-attacking part', the 'frightened self' and the 'normal self... that prays, sends bills', and is a 'carer of others'. All of these had emerged from our previous discussions and the above are her words. When trying to find an image of a 'nurturer' for herself, she was able to use an image of Jesus; he would hold her, smile, be warm and say that she needed 'care and love'. The latter image was useful in that she found it, as described, very difficult to imagine caring for herself.

On one occasion, the memory came to her of a foggy day on the beach when her father had read an animal book to her; she told me that her father had had a 'good side'. This occurred spontaneously and I had not suggested we look for good features; perhaps Susan could not accept only remembering negative things.

Narrative and metaphor

At several points in the work I gave her sheets which asked about her feelings and to express these as metaphors. When she brought the sheets to the next session we would discuss what the images might mean. Some images she gave were: an earthquake trembling; like a scared little girl; like something obstructing her throat; like a fat blob; as if 'all my insides came to my mouth' and 'I was about to throw out'. On some occasions she was able to construct a counter image; in one she said it felt as if a wall was in front of her, and for this she was able to imagine walking through this wall with Jesus holding out his hand to her.

Towards the end of the work, to reinforce the ideas we had created together, I used certain questions from Narrative Therapy (White, 2007) which were aimed at articulating her values and why she valued the new direction in her life. It was very important to articulate how harming herself was not consistent with how she saw her values and she described this as not putting love or her religion into her life.

Progress

Thirty sessions of therapy were given over approximately 12 months and then there was a follow-up after one year and a final follow-up one year and six months later. At the end of the main phase of therapy she reported making good progress in not hitting herself and not withdrawing to bed when feeling depressed. She was very well engaged in social and charitable activities and reported improving her relationship with her mother. Her scores on a test for depression suggested that she was no longer clinically depressed but she was however still somewhat anxious.

The frequency and distress of the voices improved though this fluctuated. At the very end of the main phase, however, she stated that she had had no voices for two weeks. She was seen for two further follow-up appointments and in one of them she reported a low frequency of voices during the previous weeks. In the last session she reported that she had had no voices for two months, which had been the longest time she could remember for many years.

During the assessment phase on tests for depression and anxiety her scores suggested moderate depression and quite high anxiety. In the last two follow-up meetings she was not depressed but still anxious. The work therefore seemed to have had a very large impact upon her level of depression but not on anxiety. During the phase looking at self-esteem I had asked her for percentage convictions on various statements she had made. These statements were how she saw herself and others in the world. Two scores which greatly improved were beliefs that others are 'evil' and that the world is 'vicious'. There was also a decrease in the negative belief that she ought to die because she was 'bad', and there was an increase in the statement that she was good and deserved to live.

Concluding comments

In this and the previous chapter I hoped to have shown that it is possible to do therapy with a focus on multiple states of the self for clients who experience psychosis and abuse. Such therapy may not be suitable for all clients with psychosis; furthermore, this area of work is complex and whether such therapy is effective would take extensive research. It is striking that many clients with psychosis tend to show a pattern of suffering that is similar to the kinds found in those clients who are not psychotic but who have suffered long-term traumas. I also note that it is impressive how many clients appreciate the opportunity to put their suffering in a developmental context and to work with the extreme states they find themselves experiencing in order to move forward with their lives. Finally, I hope the book as a whole helps to show how psychotic suffering is comprehensible in the context of a person's life, and that change, however difficult, is possible.

References

Arntz, A., & Weertman, A. (1999). Treatment of childhood memories: theory and practice. *Behaviour Research and Therapy*, *37*, 715–740.

Fisher, J. (2017). *Healing the fragmented selves of trauma survivors*. New York: Routledge.

Gilbert, P. (2010). *Compassion focused therapy*. Hove: Routledge.

Hayes, C., & Wijngaart, R. (2020). Imagery rescripting for childhood memories. In G. Heath, H. Startup (eds.), *Creative methods in schema therapy*. London: Routledge.

Padesky, C.A. (1994). Schema change processes in cognitive therapy. *Clinical Psychology and Psychotherapy*, *1*(5), 267–278.

Rhodes, J., & Jakes, S. (2009). *Narrative CBT for psychosis*. Hove: Routledge.

Schwartz, R.C. (1995). *Internal family systems therapy*. New York: Guilford.

Van der Hart, O., Niejenhuis, E., & Steele, K. (2006). *The haunted self: Structural dissociation and the treatment of chronic traumatisation*. New York, USA: Norton.

White, M. (2007). *Maps of narrative practice*. New York: Norton.

INDEX

3 20